In creating *Aromagick*, Diti J. Morgan has crafted a beautiful and inspiring book about the use of botanical essences in magic of many kinds. Her deep knowledge and experience of the properties of plants lays brilliantly combined with her equally deep knowledge and experience of Hindu Tantra, Western Esoterics, Mythology, and Folklore, and contemporary Neo-Paganism and Magic. She provides a rich cornucopia of spells and recipes, poetry, imagery, and lore to guide us through the seasons of the year and the many forms of magic that we can attempt at any time. A great deal of research and creativity has gone into this book, and I found much in it to surprise and delight me. I recommend this substantial and remarkable book for deep and enjoyable study, and for preservation in one's reference library.

Peter J Carroll. Stokastikos.
Southwest England, 2023.

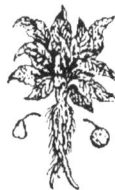

A tantalizing book which wraps Egyptian and Hindu myth, ritual, and magic around a core of expert aromatherapy and plant magic to create a complete system of magic powered by interpenetrating cycles of time. Just as the cycles of moon and sun weave together to form a calendar, so does this book twist together many strands of magic to form an eternal braid. In part one, we learn about the kalas, and ritual baths for every phase of the moon. With each phase, we deep-dive into a ritual bath. Deep and loving attention is played to the spirits of the plants on which the baths rely; each is a master-class in plant and perfume magic. In my opinion, just the bath rituals alone would easily be worth the "ticket price" for this book, but there is so much more! Nearly every chapter is bursting with poetry, essays, and juicy magical tidbits.

In part two, we expand our circle, now focusing on the eight witch's sabbats of the wheel of the year, and their relationship to the eight colors of chaos magic. Here too, Diti's depth of knowledge and joy in practice shine through. Each sabbat has a ritual bath, as well as additional material that extends, contextualizes, and tantalizes. I received the manuscript shortly before the autumn equinox, so that is where I started. The chapter opens with the powerful gnostic poem "Thunder, Perfect Mind" from the Nag Hammadi manuscripts, continues with an invocation of the Egyptian fertility goddess Ipet, moves on to a short essay about the magical virtues of the color blue, and its relation to the season, and then provides an essay by noted scholar of Egyptian magic (and Diti's husband) Mogg Morgan about Ma'at, the Egyptian deification of Divine Balance. The chapter concludes, as each does, with an amazing dreamy bath recipe – this one centered on blue lotus, chamomile, jasmine, frankincense, and bergamot. Just listing the ingredients is enough to make me swoon at their intoxicating fragrance! All of that is just one chapter of this fascinating book! I can't wait to continue working with it throughout the year.

Sara L Mastros author of *The Sorcery of Solomon:*
A Guide to The 44 Planetary Pentecals of the Magician king

Aromagick

A Scentual Guide to the Lunar Essence of the Kalas and the Eight Colours of Magick

Diti J. Morgan

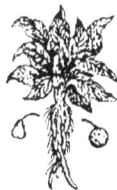

To Mogg
Love and do what you will

Disclaimer

Take appropriate precautions and keep your wits about you. The information in this book should not be used as a substitute for professional advice. Neither the author nor publisher can be held responsible for any loss, claim or damage arising out of the use, or misuse of the suggestions made.

Contents

Acknowledgments

I am greatly indebted to my friend Ana Jones for her constant support and counsel throughout this venture. My heart overflows with appreciation for always being there whenever I needed a shoulder. Marina (Li Chun) Lin deserves special recognition for her kindness and generosity, radiant smiles, and wonderful Chinese tea ceremonies. My sincere thanks go out to Elizabeth Ashley for sharing her knowledge of combining vetiver and palmarosa to bring the aroma of beetroot to fruition. Her advice was invaluable. Lastly, a thank you goes to William Breeze, head of the OTO, for his aid in clearing up certain queries concerning Liber Resh.

My heartfelt thanks go out to Mike Magee for his extensive research, expertise and translations of the Tantric texts, which have ignited a passionate interest in the Kalas within me. I must also extend my gratitude to Gregory Peters whose insightful observations concerning the nature of the Kalas and especially Ugraprabha have been invaluable.

I am immensely grateful to Roy Morgan for supplying the stunning photographs used for the cover of this publication. Many thanks are due to Peter Carroll, Michael Kelly, Jan Fries, Jason Read, and Egyptologist Dora Goldsmith. Their input has been a highly inspirational force throughout my work on this project.

Many thanks to the MorganWitches clan for witnessing my journey of becoming.

XEPHER

Introduction

Smell

The faculty or power of perceiving odours or scents by means of the organs in the nose. As in "a highly developed sense of smell" (Oxford English Dictionary)

Ever since I was little, I had a strong desire to smell everything around me. I remember my mother telling me that it took forever to get me ready because I insisted on smelling each piece of clothing I was given, even down to my socks and shoes. Growing up on a farm exposed me to various scents that helped me form connections with animals, plants, and the environment. Despite the potent and unappealing aroma of goats, it brings back fond memories of early mornings and tiring yet fulfilling days of herding them. I gained a wealth of knowledge from these creatures, and my admiration for them is reflected in several of the fragrance oils I created and described in this publication. In addition, the fragrance of fresh hay and clean straw takes me back to the stables during mealtime, a cherished aroma — the sweet, smooth, and balsamic-like scent of a horse's nose. This is a secret scent that equestrians are intimately familiar with and will recognize instantly upon reading these words. Moreover, we must not overlook the musky scent of rabbits, the pungent aroma of the chicken coop, and the milky scent of newborn puppies.

Surrounding the farm are groves of oranges and lemons, as well as fields of barley. One can observe the changing of the seasons through their sense of smell. The delightful aroma of orange and lemon blossoms on autumn evenings lifts the spirits and fills one's heart with joy. The sweet fragrance of oranges signals the arrival of winter, accompanied by the earthy scents of damp soil and moist fields. The fresh and verdant green barley is a sign that spring has arrived, bringing with it a profusion of wildflowers. As June draws to a close, most of the wildflowers have withered away and the air begins to feel hot and dry. July and August are characterised by the combined scents of hot soil, dry plants, perspiring bodies, and a refreshing breeze from the beach.

My fascination with scents and aromas led me to study aromatherapy. Working with essential oils for so many years, I began to believe that plants are sentient. According to Daniel Shulke's *Ars Philtron*: …"Fresh material, especially that which proceeds directly into the menstruum secondes after harvest, possesses an undeniably greater level of vivified spirit than that material which has been severed from its parent plant and laid on a drying rack for a week or more." …"When creating Flower Essences, living plant portions are essential."

Odorant molecules found in essential oils are responsible for the smells we perceive. These molecules stimulate sensory nerve cells located at the top of the nasal cavity, which then send impulses to the olfactory bulb in the brain's smell centre. The olfactory bulb recognizes smells as part of the limbic system, whose function is to process and regulate emotions and memory while also dealing with sexual stimulation, learning, behaviour and motivation. Essential oils are volatile (easily evaporated) compounds extracted from plants and give each essential oil its characteristic essence. The oils capture the plant's scent and flavour, or "essence." Essential oils are obtained mainly through steam or water distillation or other methods, such as cold pressing/expression and solvent extraction.

My aromatherapy teacher, the late Sheila Brooke, taught me how to connect with the spirits of the oils and their true essence. She used to say: "Think of them (the essential oils) like they are Genies in bottles. Always approach with respect, keep an open mind and consider carefully the information you want to obtain from them." As a diligent learner, I quickly became acquainted with the volatile pure essences. As I continued to experiment with both single and blended essences, I observed that the fragrances I used had a noticeable impact on my overall mood, for instance, a single essence or a blend of essential oils can change, trigger or enhance various emotions and sensations such as irritation, stress, depression, apathy, happiness, sensuality, relaxation and stimulation. With time, my understanding of the complexity of those precious volatile compounds evolved, and with it, the channels of communication grew deeper between myself and those fragrant Genies in bottles.

Definition: I use the word essence as a reference to the sentient consciousness of essential oils.

As I learned and experimented more, I realized that I wasn't just dealing with plant chemistry and molecules, but the pure essence of the essential oil I was studying. Years of working as an aromatherapist practitioner taught me that taking a meditative and ritualistic approach while handling essential oils can elevate my blending skills to a higher level. My sessions with the clients became somewhat of a "shamanic journey" — a kind of soul retrieval of both myself and the client. An integral part of my work as an aromatherapy practitioner was prescribing personalized tailored bath blends. My experiments with different essential oil blends led me to the understanding that when mixing/blending certain essences together, something unique and magical can happen. It is not just that our mood is changing, but there is a shift in our consciousness and with the right atmosphere, a meditative kind of ritual — a bath in our case, we can enter through the doors of perception and experience altered states of mind, albeit subtle ones. Just to make it clear, the journey with the essences is an initiatory and subtle one and not a full-blown psychedelic trip. This is the same with certain blends such as those given in the Eight Witches Sabbaths section. This type of experience will usually follow with a flood of insights, new ideas, occult revelations and personal gnosis.

Although aromatherapy is a big part of my life, this book has been written about the magical aspect of aromatics and their essences. I chose not to write about the chemistry and physiological benefits of the essential oils in the book. Information on those subjects is vast and wide. For further reading on Aromatherapy, please check the bibliography section at the end of the book.

Any aromatherapist who is worth their salt, or (essential) oil in our case, will realise pretty soon in their practice, that working with essential oils can be very similar to writing spells, invocations, incantations and conjurations. So if you asked me what came first, aromatherapy or magic, I will probably say that in my case, both evolved simultaneously.

As part of my initiation into AMOOKOS, an East-West Kaula Mystery School, I dedicated a big chunk of my studies to learning about the Kala sequence. Kala, meaning part, perhaps "lunar perfume or flower". The Hindu erotic texts, for instance, the Ananga Ranga (Play of the Bodiless One) seem to use a system based on the 30-day lunar cycle. Each Kala represents the daily phase of the moon and part of our body. The concept of 'Lunar Perfume' is speculative and from Kenneth Grant's *Outside the Circles of Time*, so you won't find it listed as a meaning in any dictionary. But given that the concept is applied to parts of the body, it seems to work perfectly with the Ananga Ranga system mentioned above. Each Kala corresponds to a different phase of the moon, and a different body part. It didn't take long for the concept of 'Lunar Perfume' to evolve to a whole new way of working with the Kala sequence.

For many moons, on the 3rd day of the new moon, my head was filled with images of Nityaklinna. The common theme of the images was water and fluidity. Sometimes she was coming out of the river, on others, she was in the rain or covered with sweat and some kind of red paste smeared all over her body and face. I must confess that those striking images and visions were the inspiration for writing this book.

In the second part of the book, I deal with the Eight Witches Sabbaths of the Ritual Year and how they resonate with the Eight Magics and the corresponding colours and scented essences. According to Peter Carroll's *Liber Kaos* — "Our perceptual and conceptual apparatus creates a fourfold division of matter into the space, time, mass, and energy tautology. Similarly, our instinctual drives create an eightfold division of magic. The eight forms of magic are conveniently denoted by colours having emotional significance". (p. 107)

In the magical system of the Chaos Craft current (check out *Chaos Craft* by Julian Vayne & Steve Dee), the eight magics and their colours are assigned to each of the witch's sabbaths. As a witch initiated to the Chaos Craft current, I was unable to ignore the connection of colours and essences with each cycle of the year's wheel.

The chapters dealing with the witch's sabbaths and the eight colours of magick, will take you on an initiatory journey and connect you to the corresponding energies of each sabbath. I captured the distinctive signature and characteristics of each colour and essence, in a series of unique perfume oils, corresponding to each of the Eight Witches Sabbats. Each perfume oil can be used also as a stand-alone initiatory or invocation oil, according to the energies it corresponds with. For example, Red Magick perfume oil can be used to invoke or initiate any of the following: vibration, glow, determination and assertiveness, sex, breaking habits, purification, protection, aggression and strength, and any deity which is associated with the colour red.

Each perfume oil is a portal to one of the eight magics. Those of you who will dare enter it with the aid of one of the perfumes might discover that each portal leads to a magical realm and a scentual gnosis, that at times is much too personal to write about.

May your journey be colourful and scentual

Diti J Morgan
Red Magick 2023

Part I
The Kala Cycle

"Who am I, and what shall be the sign? So she answered him, bending down, a lambent flame of blue, all-touching, all penetrant, her lovely hands upon the black earth, & her lithe body arched for love, and her soft feet not hurting the little flowers: Thou knowest! And the sign shall be my ecstasy, the consciousness of the continuity of existence, the omnipresence of my body." *Liber Al* 1:26

Aroma is an invocation

1. Kalas
Essence of the Lunar Flowers

Kala, means part, perhaps also a "lunar perfume or flower". These mysterious but extremely important principles, derived from esoteric Hinduism, were related to the cosmic tides of the moon, those that ebb and flow during the course of a lunar month. Though important, it was not until recent times, that this material became better understood. They were first described in the Tantrik systems and texts, as components of a person's psychic anatomy, alongside other more well known concepts such as the serpent power kundalini, the psychic centres or chakras, and the serpent like streams of energy, known as nadis. They are therefore elements in what we in the west might call the alchemical body.

Knowledge of the kalas found its way into the western esoteric tradition but the information was very cryptic and limited. It became known that the Hindus envisioned the body as a microcosm of the world, in effect the kalas representing cycle of the moon within each of our bodies:

> "An individual is a microcosm of the universe as all material and spiritual phenomena of the universe are present in the individual and all those present in the individual are also contained in the universe." (Charaka, ancient Hindu physician)

This has huge implications for the techniques of the body. The Hindu erotic texts, for instance, the Hindu *Ananga Ranga* ('Play of the Bodiless One') seem to use this system based on the 30-day lunar cycle. Each Kala represents the daily phase of the moon and a body part. In the west there is an important style of magick and esoteric lore which has come to be known as the Typhonian, a darkly erotic tradition ultimately derived from the magical religion of ancient Egypt and its passionate, erotic deity Seth-Typhon and his companions. One thing for sure, in this typhonian magick the lunar sequence always features very strongly, one way or another.

For example, the concept of 'Lunar Perfume' is taken from Kenneth Grant's *Outside the Circles of Time*. It is not exactly listed in the Sanskrit dictionary where the concept is only applied to parts of the body. However, it seems to fit perfectly with the system of the 'Ananga Ranga' mentioned above.

The moon rules over water and the cycle of the moon is what rules the tides. Our body is constituted of 75% water thus it's hardly surprising to find that we, like all beings, are strongly affected by the cycle of the moon. The Kala system is best understood through a month-long journey of focus and meditation practices throughout the body. For over two decades, I have dedicated myself to aromatherapy, and in recent years this has been enriched by exploring the Kalas. It didn't take long for me to recognize the correlation between them, and with every lunar cycle, I was able to gain an increasingly profound understanding of their relationship as my body became more in harmony with its natural rhythms. Like a dial on a clock that marks seconds and minutes, the Kalas represent the moon's motions during its monthly cycle. I find it very helpful to visualize the Kalas as tiny movements or motions in the endless cycle of the Ouroboros serpent. Its pulsating body, ever ready to shed its skin, ever-changing. In my search for understanding the Kalas, I found that if I placed an imaginary cardinal cross inside a circle, it made it so much easier to understand the essence of each Kala. My four cardinal Kalas are:

Kamesvari – new moon,

Duti/Tavrita – first quarter,

Amrita/Kali – full moon and

Ugra/Ugraprabha – last quarter.

Going deeper, you can orient your work around the eight Sabbats of the wheel of the year, appreciating the Kala that resides over each Sabbat and enhances the energies of that day and night. You will find that each month and year, the Kalas will vary slightly as the cycle of the moon is in constant motion.

From Shakti to Kali

Each lunar day is said to have its unique magical quality.

The following poem is inspired by a couple's intimate exploration of one cycle of the Kalas.

Shakti
That's how you named me
And yes why not
I am beautiful
And wise
Like Shakti
I am kind
funny
sexy
and happy

I love
and I am loved
In the mornings

when I wake up
by your side
two suns rising in my eyes
Shining light so bright
I can see your body
sparkle with golden dust
I could see your heart
melting into the stones
When we kissed under the
Golden dawn
For 15 days and nights
We are shining bright
Happy
Dancing
Kissing
Telling little love stories
to each other
The stories of Kameshvari and her
ankle bracelet
Duti The impossible girl messenger
and ChitraMalini
The bright one
The full one
The one who initiates her twin sister
Kali
Tonight is the 15th night of
sweet love
Long kisses
Passion and desires
I am Shakti

The lady of desire
Messenger of love
Bright garland
The kiss of life
I am Shakti
My eyes shine like
Two bright suns
but if you look closely
You will see
Two black suns rising inside
I am Kali
I am the dark one
You can only see me
when the moon is full
I am Kali
My eyes are two black suns
Which will darken your days
And blacken your sights
I am Kali
I'll spread my darkness
Slowly slowly
You will not even notice
When it touches your heart
But on the Seventh-day
When a black tear will
Drop on your shoulder

You will know only confusion
and darkness
Your heart will be broken

Only then you will know

That The Terrible,

The Formidable

Has been awakened

I am Ugra

I am darkness

From now till the end of the cycle

You will know only darkness

The night sky will grow darker and darker

You can only see the artificial stars

I am Ugra

I am a nightcrawler

I will dim the lights

In your heart

One by one

Till you won't

Be able to see

Only darkness

Only me

And at the end of your cycle

You will not

Be able to tell

Was it, Mita or

Mahakali

I am alive!

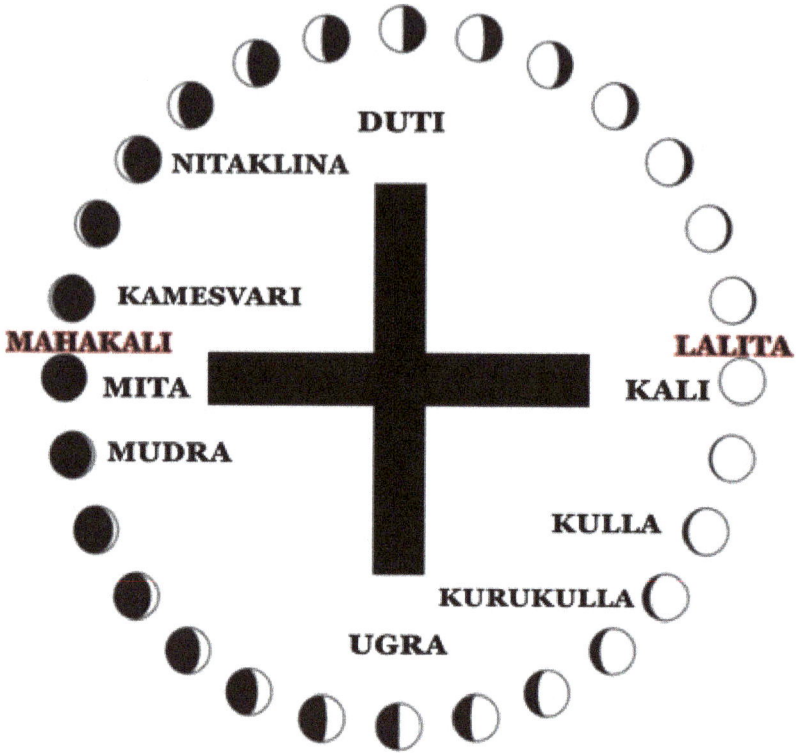

DUTI
NITAKLINA
KAMESVARI
MAHAKALI
MITA
MUDRA
LALITA
KALI
KULLA
KURUKULLA
UGRA

The moon cycle is made of two different sequences. The first is calculated from the new moon to the full moon and is associated with the waxing moon, the 'light' moon and Shakti. The second sequence is known as the 'dark or Kali sequence' and it corresponds with the waxing moon. It is calculated from the full moon to the new moon. The Sixteen Kala will be celebrated on the full moon and on the night of the dark moon. Each Kalas seems to be arranged in couples, which is most apparent to notice on the four cardinal points (see the Kala Mandala table).

Duti/Tvarita at the waxing moon
Amrita/Kali at the full moon

Ugra/UgraPrabha at the waning moon
Kameshvari on the new moon.

It seems that each of the Kala couples is sharing similar energy and essence. However, the first one to arrive (say Ugra), set herself in the new phase of the rising moon, symbolising the decline of the Kala that is just gone. While the second Kala (UgraPrabha), sat in the day, symbolically opening the way to the rising of the next Kala.

The Kala Mandala

Here follows a summary in a form of a table (a "mandala") of the entire system of kalas and their corresponding qualities.

Light Half (Shukla Paksha)

Light Half (Shukla Paksha)

Lunar Day	Nitya Goddesses	Translation	Body Locus	From Drawing	Insights	Essential oils
1	Kameshvari	Kāmeśvari is the consort of Kamesvara (one of the forms of Siva). Lady of Desire 'She who gives Her breasts to Kamesvara in return for the gem of love He bestows on Her'. 'She who gives rise to Ganesa by a glance at the face of Kamesvara.' 'Kamesvara prana nadi'- She who is the very life of Kamesvara, her consort. Devi is the vital nerve (prana nadi) of Siva.	Foot & Ankle fire	Foot Element of fire	Holding a Kapala	Camphor (as Ishtar) Spikenard Clary sage *** Clary Sage and Spikenard can be combined in one blend; however, Camphor oil should **only** be used in a diffuser or an oil burner.
2	Bhagamalini	Flower Yoni	Knee represents 'moving forward' & creativity	Ankle fire	The creative womb of the goddess. Holding a Kapala	Calendula Bergamot Geranium
3	Nitya Klinna	She who is eternally wet with love	Yoni water	Knee fire	Holding a Kapala	Geranium
4	Bherunda	Molten Gold/The Terrible?	Pubis earth	Groin earth		Vetiver Patchouli
5	Vahni Vasini	Dweller in Fire	Hip air	Yoni water	Time to Surrender to the growing light and power of the moon	Clary sage Ylang--Ylang Lavender
6	Mahavajravari	Great Goddess of the Vajra	Side air	Hip air	Mahavajra manifests the energy of protection and the removal of obstacles.	Eucalyptus. Fennel Lavender Peppermint

					Making space for new light, ideas and energy. And expanding our knowledge.	
7	Dyutidhara Sivduti	The Messenger	Breast air	Navel fire	Duti is full of light and splendour. She has an aura of light.	Rose
8	Tvarita	Swift One	Armpit air	Lower Breast air		Rose, 'Venusian Dragon' perfume oil Lemon Balm
9	Kulasundari	Beautiful Mound	Shoulder air	Upper breast air		Lemon Lemongrass Lavender
10	Nitya Nitya	She who is eternal, 'the everlasting goddess'	Neck air	Shoulder air	'There is nothing eternal' Holding a Kapala	Abramelin oil is a reminder that nothing is eternal but magic. Baphomet oil
11	Nilapataka	Falling Sapphire	Chin ether	Neck air	Holding a Kapala	Lavender
12	Vijaya	Victorious Bow. One with special knowledge "The auspicious hour"	Lips ether	Cheek air		Sage Lavender
13	Sarvamangala	All Auspicious	Cheek air	Lips ether	Holding a Kapala	Sage Lily of the valley
14	Jvalamālini	Fire Garland. "She who has taken position at the centre of the fortress of fire created by the goddess"	Eyes The element of fire.	Eyes fire	Jvalamalin is the one who throws flames all around. The full moon is nearly here, and she is preparing us for the fire rite of the eternal fire of truth. For the state of enlightenment	Ruthvah oil Jitterybug perfume oil

15	ChitraMālini	Bright Garland, She who is wearing garlands. ChitraMalini symbolises the boons of bloom, purification & knowledge.	Forehead Third eye fire	Forehead. Malini, as the Ganga, represents purification. She is the fiery aspect of the water and creation.	Garland of red flowers, the Garland of waves of Ganga. Garland of the 51 letters of the Sanskrit.	Neroli, Orange, Juniper, Abramelin oil.
16	Lalita Amrita-kala - The full moon	Sometimes Sadakhya 'She who is the Ultimate Truth'	Eternal/ True Face	The five elements.	From Gopinath Kaviraj's introduction ? - "The sixteenth Kala called Sadakhya should be viewed as one with Lalita or the Supreme Deity Herself. In other words, one has to feel that what appears is nothing but an expression of what exists eternally" -Lokanath	Twilight. The Lily came to bloom in the early hours of the morning, just after the dawn of the full moon day. In the dark of the moon. Clary Sage will help us to see what is ahead of us, invoke our dreams and new ideas and expand our vision and set us with clarity into a new beginning of a new cycle. Holding a Kapala. For the full moon: White Water Lily- (Lotus). Jasmine. Opoponax For the new moon: clary sage

Dark Half (Krishna or Kali Paksha)

Dark Half (Krishna or Kali Paksha)

1	Kali	Dark	Forehead Third eye	Element of fire	Holding a Kapala	Red Hibiscus
2	Kapalini	Skull Girl	Eyes - element of fire	There is a female Kapalika cult, the female devotee who smeared herself in the ashes of her lover's funeral pyre. (see Ghatasaptasai. Kapalini, a Yakshini who provides daily food, clothing and money, tells the future and bestows long life, but she seldom becomes a partner in sexual practices.	Skull represents The concept of being in our body and not so much in the head takes the focus from the intellect into the physical. The skull also represents the vessel of transcendence of death. Dawn to midnight	Jasmine Basil, Bergamot, Copal. Orange. Abramelin oil. Baphomet oil
3	Kulla	Ancestral	Cheek air	She who is the deity in the kulas, the essence of the universe and the essence of knowledge	Kula is defined as the state in which all thoughts of plurality based on the sense of time, place, cause, action, and effect dissolve completely "All is one" "אין מים" A country or the home.	Spikenard, Lavender
4	KuruKulla	Tribal	Lips ether	"She who is the cause of knowledge"	Kurukulla Holding a Kapala	White Lotus. Black magick oil
5	Varodhini	She sets her face against the world	Chin ether	An apsara, a spirit of the clouds and moisture		Clary sage Lavender Star Anis

6	VipraChitta	Seething-Mind, Sagacious Mind	Neck Element of air	The word vipra has lots of interesting meanings, including to tremble in a shamanic way. But here it is usually translated as "passionate mind" or "one who loves passion" perhaps one whose mind is swift-moving with thought, hence sagacious	Morning Holding a Kapala	Black magick oil
7	Ugra	The Terrible, formidable	Shoulder air	'The Hungry One' The eternal hunger for knowledge	Midnight till dawn. Star of David Yantra. "She who brings us to the other shore"	Blue lotus
8	UgraPrabha	radiant (Prabha) Ugra	Armpit air	Holding a Kapala	The Blue lotus blooms till midday	Blue lotus
9	DipaNitya	Eternal Light	Breast air	Holding a Kapala		Lemon Balm
10	NilaNitya	Blue Light	Side air			Lotus Lily of the valley
11	Ghana	'The deep dark one', Darkness, dark colour, Dence, striker, destroyer	Hip Element of air			Galbanum
12	Balaka	"Strong one" appears in twilight dreams	Pubis Element of air	Groin air		Galbanum
13	Matra	Mother & Measure	Yoni Element of water	Holding a Kapala		Geranium Tuberose
14	Mudra	Gesture, body, magical	Knee Element of fire			Abramelin Oil Red Magick oil

15	Mita	The Measurer	Foot Element of fire	"She who resides inside the kula, between the measurer and the measured in the form of the measure". Holding a Kapala	Mita represents the end of the cycle that started with Kula, she has the measures of the time, place, cause, action and effect. With those measures, we can go on and start a new cycle.	Helichrysum Calendula
16	Mahakali The Dark Moon			Holding a Kapala	Past, Future and Present Here and now	Red Hibiscus

2. Kameswari

As a new lunar month begins, the energy of the New Moon invites us to embrace new beginnings and renewal. Kameswari's footsteps serve as a guide for us to tune into this energy and start fresh each month. By focusing on our intentions, ideas, and dreams, we can transform them into creative manifestations.

From *The Thousand Names of the Divine Mother* by Sri Lalita Sahasranama, we learn that Kameswari's name means "The Lady of Love and Desire". She is garlanded with red hibiscus and gold jewellery, and a golden skullcup (Kapala). Sometimes she will appear holding a golden sword, bow and arrows. Kameswari guides us, towards the potential opportunities that may arise in the upcoming month. As Her name implies, 'Lady of Desire', it seems that by focusing on our genuine aspirations, we may be able to mould the future days in accordance with our objectives and ambitions. Kameswari corresponds with the essence of Clary Sage. As its name suggests, Clary is the oil of clarity, clear thinking and clear visions. Using Clary sage on the new moon will direct Kameswari's essence and energy, our way. A few drops in the ritual bath will help us to open up to changes, new ideas and new perceptions. Will clear our minds and make space for new visions and dreams.

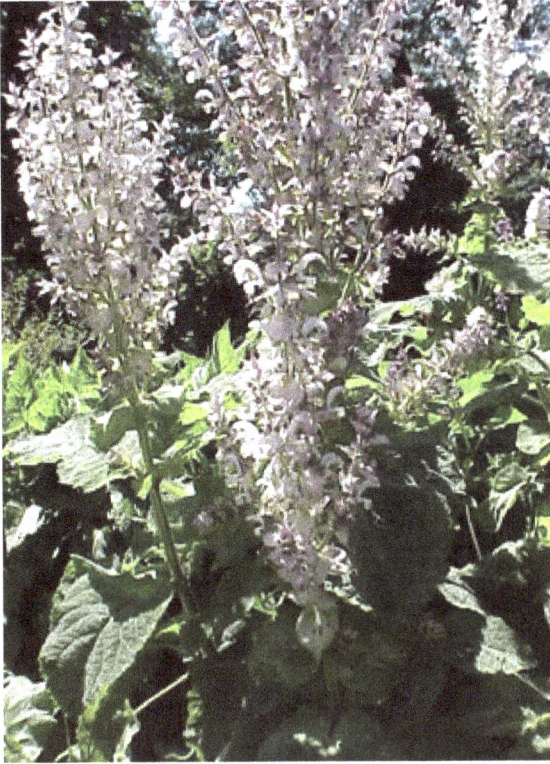

Clary Sage, *Salvia sclarea*

(Photo courtesy of wiki commons.wikimedia.org/wiki/File:Salvia,sclarea3.jpg)

Salvia Sclara/Clary sage is a perennial herb that grows up to a metre high and has large, hairy leaves and small blue-purple flowers. It is native to southern Europe but is cultivated worldwide, especially in the Mediterranean. It is closely related to garden sage. If you are experiencing feelings of depression, stress, insomnia, or tension, Clary Sage has the ability to soothe your nerves and promote relaxation in both your mind and body. Moreover, it possesses anti-depressant properties that can uplift your mood and offer advantageous effects on the female reproductive system, aiding with various issues ranging from premenstrual tension to menopause.

Clary sage essential oil has a soothing effect on both the mind and body, promoting restful sleep and vivid dreams. It is also linked to feelings of euphoria and is often associated with enhanced vision. Additionally, it is utilized to clear both the physical and spiritual "third eye" of those who practice clairvoyance or divination. It is said to boost one's spirits and facilitate detachment from emotionally challenging situations, providing a clearer perspective. Some people use it to enter a trance state or experience euphoria, which is why it is occasionally used as an aphrodisiac.

New Moon Bath ritual

Prepare your oil blend in a small bowl, with one tablespoon of sea salt and about 6-9 drops of Clary Sage essential oil. When your bath is full, add the blend into the bath and make the figure eight in the water while focusing on your intentions and prayers and offering yourself (by getting into the water) to the spirit of the oil. Once you're in the bath, let your body relax in the water, close your eyes, take a few deep breaths and inhale the scent of the oil while listening to your guided meditation or saying your chosen mantra. Repeat the mantra as many times as it feels right and works for you. Using a mantra can serve as a catalyst for taking your first conscious step into a new cycle. Once you sense a shift or breakthrough, you may choose to continue meditating or express your gratitude. Then, with a symbolic step forward, proceed with the remainder of your day or evening.

Chandra (Moon) Gayatri mantra:
om kshira-putraya vidmahe
amrita-tattvaya dhimahi
tanno chandra prachodayat
I bow down to Lord Chandra, holder of the lotus.
Who shines in the brilliant colour of gold.

May Lord Chandra illuminate my intellect
and shed light on my path.

When a bath is not an option, inhale the oil while listening to the mantra/ meditation. Once the mantra is over, utter the license to depart (say thanks and put the Clary Sage bottle away).

***Excessive inhalation of the Clary sage oil might cause headaches!

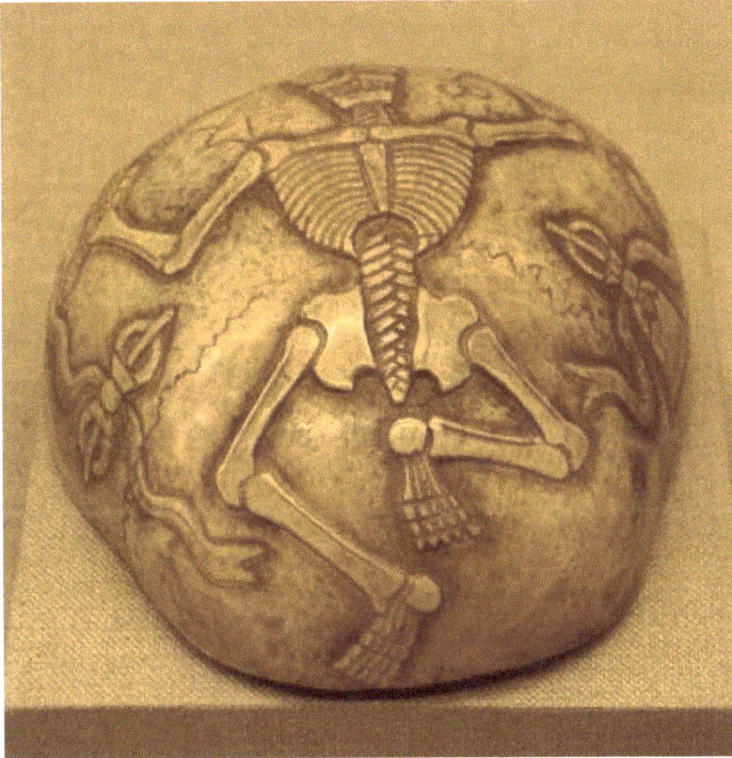

The Kapala
(Photo courtesy of wiki commons.wikimedia.org/wiki/File:Kapala,skull,cup.jpg)

The Kapala, which means "skull" in Sanskrit, serves as a ritual tool or bowl in both Hindu Tantra and Buddhist Tantra (Vajrayana). The use of kapalas in higher tantric meditation aims to achieve a transcendental state of mind.

To prepare the kapala for tantric ceremonies and rituals, sacred mantras were written on the interior of the cranium, while the exterior of the skull was adorned with sacred and magical syllables invoking the deity's body, speech, and mind. This was done to purify the contents and ensure that the kapala was appropriate for ritual use. Kapalas were frequently adorned with intricate metal bases and covers as a way to remind individuals of the fleeting nature of the body and the significance of letting go. Using human remains as a ceremonial vessel served as a symbol of impermanence and detachment. It was thought that the vital energy of the deceased individual to whom the skull once belonged, was contained within the Kapala, which rendered it a powerful object imbued with magic. Magical and spiritual rituals frequently utilized the skull cup, particularly in the "inner offering" ceremony. During this rite, the practitioner would envision the skull as their severed head and pour their "internal poison" into it. These poisons or obstacles were represented by the five elixirs (or the five taboos). They each represented form, feelings, perceptions, karmic impulses, and consciousness. The next stage of the rite involves the practitioner invoking their chosen tantric deity into themselves while visualizing the content of the skull cup brought to a boiling point. This transforms the internal poison into the divine nectar.

There are 32 unique energies that make up the Kala cycle, representing each day of a month. Sixteen of these Kalas are shown holding a Kapala, eight of them are part of the Shakti or light cycle, and the other eight belong to the Kali or dark cycle of the lunar cycle. The Kalas represent a powerful symbol of transformation, providing us with an opportunity to identify and overcome any internal barriers that may be hindering our progress. By engaging in a personal and distinctive practice of inner offering during the phases of the moon, we have the potential to bring about a significant metamorphosis within ourselves.

To all intent and purposes, obtaining a human skull for use in your rites is prohibited for most people like us, it's too expensive, too anti-social and just wrong. In the Hindu Tantra tradition, it is common and even advisable to substitute a coconut for the human skull cup as the vessel of transformation.

The skull-cup bearers are:

Kali
Kapalini
Kurukulla
Vipracitta
Ugraprabha
Dipa
Matra (menstrual blood)
Mita
Kamesvari
Bhagmalini
Nityaklinna
Nitya
Nilapataka
Sarvamangala
Lalita
Mahakali (dark moon)

3. NityaKlinna
Geranium – Fluidity

Moon phase – 3 days into the new moon
NityaKlinna – 'She who is eternally wet with love'

For many moons, on the 3rd day of the new moon, my head was filled with images of Nityaklinna. The common theme of the images was of water and fluidity. Sometimes she was coming out of the river, on others, she was in the rain or covered with sweat and some kind of red paste smeared all over her body and face. I must say that those striking images and visions inspired writing this book.

According to The *Tantraraja*, Nityaklinna, is restless with desire, smeared with red sandal paste, wears red clothes, smiles, has a half-moon on her head, and holds a noose, goad, cup and makes the mudra dispelling fear. The Dakshinamurti Samhita's image is similar except that she holds a noose, a goad, and a skull. Her face is bathed in sweat and her eyes move with desire. She is holding a cup that always overflows with fluids which might suggest her role as the teacher of the mysteries of the water. Her cup could also suggest the ever-flowing nectar of the goddess. The noose and the goad suggesting fluidity and motion and ever moving forward, navigating the current of nature and the flow of water in rivers, lakes and oceans along with the tide of the moon.

Working with the Kalas has helped me tune my body to the essences and phases of the moon. Synchronicity has become a big part of my daily life with each cycle of the moon. During one moon cycle, I dreamt of NityaKlinna emerging from the water like in Botticelli's 'The Birth of Venus'. This dream gave me an interesting insight that Geranium must be the essence of Nityaklinna. Geranium is related to the water element and resonates with the planet Venus, just like NityaKlinna, 'she who is eternally wet with love'. Its magical uses are to promote happiness, well-being and protection and regeneration, which corresponds with her hand mudra.

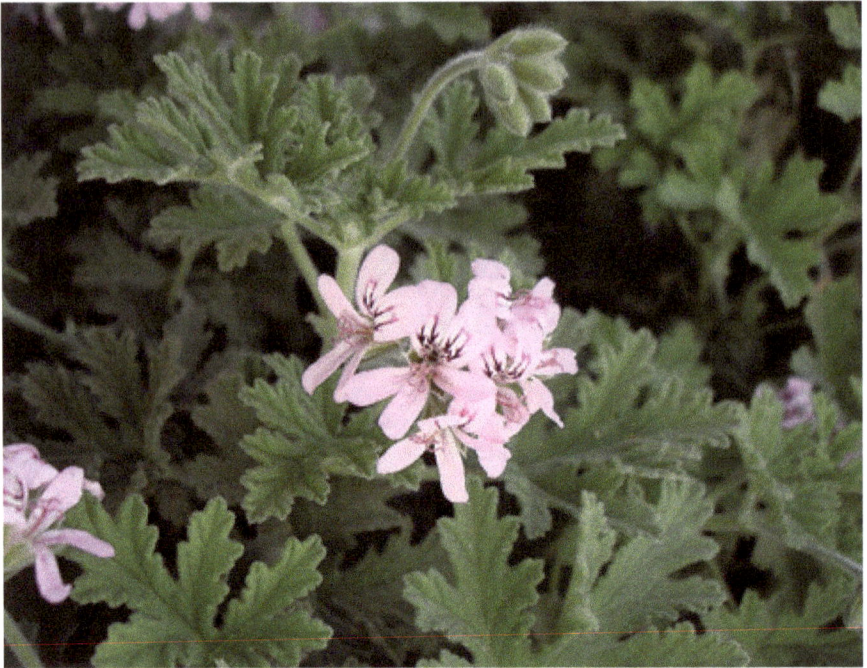

Geranium, Pelargonium graveolens
(Photo courtesy of wiki commons.wikimedia.org/wiki/
File:Pelargonium,graveolens,A1.jpg)

The shrub called Geranium is known for its small pink flowers and can grow up to a metre high. It is originally from South Africa and is now being cultivated in Egypt, China, and the Reunion Islands for essential oil production. Throughout history, Geranium has been utilized for a wide range of applications including treating Acne, bruises, burns, dermatitis, eczema, haemorrhoids, oily complexion, mature skin, mosquito repellent, oedema, poor circulation, PMT and menopausal problems, as well as stress-related conditions.

The scent's fresh greenness and sweet aroma can have a positive impact on our mental state, opening our hearts and uplifting our spirits. The gentle fragrance's lightness can help balance and calm an anxious person. When I was first starting out with my aromatherapy practice, I would host a series of house parties focused on aromatherapy. These events were a great way to showcase my products and promote my business, which included selling essential oils and beauty products. I used to love passing around a bottle of Geranium at my aromatherapy parties. It was amazing to see how the atmosphere in the room would shift from a formal business gathering to a more relaxed and intimate event. Everyone seemed to let their guard down and become more open and interested in the presentation and products. Plus, the sweet aroma just made people smile and feel at ease. Even after 25 years, whenever I want to create a positive and relaxing environment, my go-to choice is always Geranium. Its sweet fragrance has the ability to uplift and put everyone at ease, just like it did back in the days of my aromatherapy parties.

Through a simple party trick, I discovered the amazing power of essential oils to enhance moods and alter minds. This discovery ignited a lifelong journey of exploration, which you will witness in the upcoming chapters.

Geranium is ruled by the planet Venus and is associated with the element of water. Like Venus, Nityaklinna honours us with love, sensuality, beauty, youth, creativity, protection and the fluidity of life itself. She is the first prominent light of the new moon and from now on, the light of the Shakti cycle will grow stronger and brighter every night till its peak on the night of the full moon. Geranium has a stimulating effect on our circulation improving our blood and lymph flow. Maintaining the efficient flow of body fluids is crucial for good health and mental well-being as we are predominantly (60-75%) made of water. The essence of a happy and healthy life lies in the flow of water, which is sensual and creative. Nityaklinna's teachings stress the importance of not allowing the water within us to become stagnant. Following a period of almost three days of darkness, Nityaklinna emerges and creates the first ripple in the flowing river of the lunar cycle.

Ritual bath

The practice of Ritual Bath holds great religious or magical importance, as it involves the use of water to spiritually cleanse or anoint the initiate. The particular ritual may call for the participant to fully submerge themselves in water, or to simply wash their hands, face, or feet, or even receive a symbolic sprinkling of water. For instance, in Judaism, a pool of natural water called Mikvah (also spelt Mikveh or Miqwe) is used for ritual purification. The Mishna, which is the Jewish code of law, provides extensive instructions on the proper water requirements and the amount of water necessary for the cleansing ritual. In the past, Mikvahs were so important to Jewish communities that they would go as far as selling their synagogues to fund their construction. Water has many symbolic associations, including with the unconscious mind, intuition, and emotions. It represents life, purity, fertility, and movement. The transformative power of water is evident in its ability to change from liquid to solid to vapour. While bathing rituals can take place in bodies of water like the sea, rivers, streams, lakes, or ponds, many of the rituals in this book are designed for the bathroom, where individuals can create their own private sanctuary and fully immerse themselves in the water. When I prepare for my ritual, the bathroom becomes my sacred space. I make sure it is clean and pure, with all mirrors sparkling clean to invite clear visions. During my Aromagick rituals, the bath itself becomes the altar, and the water is the alchemical vessel for metamorphosis. I add all the necessary elements for transformation into the vessel, along with my humble offerings. This is where the true magic happens.

To begin the ritual, fill the bath with water and adjust the temperature to your liking. While I prefer hot water, it's important that you choose a comfortable temperature since you'll be soaking in the bath for at least 15 minutes. When the bath is full to your satisfaction, add your offering to the water. Aromagick bath offerings consist mainly of essential oils, salts, dry flowers and herbs. Nevertheless, the most crucial aspect of the ritual is you. When we immerse ourselves in the vessel of transformation, we offer ourselves to the water and undergo profound enlightenment and transformation.

As you prepare to take a bath, try making a gentle figure-eight motion with your hand as you allow any worries or concerns to float away while asking for guidance, insights or protection. After getting into the warm water, let your body fully unwind and relax. Take a moment to close your eyes, take deep breaths, and inhale the scent of your chosen essential oil. For added relaxation, you may want to listen to a guided meditation of your choice to let go of any stress or tension. I find it helpful to curate a playlist that lasts around 15-25 minutes. I usually start with some soothing music for 5-10 minutes, then follow it up with 10 minutes of guided meditation, and finish with another 5-10 minutes of tranquil music. Once the music ends, you'll know it's time to conclude your bath routine.

You can use the following description of the Kala as a visual focus meditation while taking your ritual bath:

> "Nityaklinna, is restless with desire, smeared with red sandal paste, wears red clothes, smiles, has a half-moon on her head, and holds a noose, goad, and cup and makes the mudra dispelling fear."

Nityaklinna ritual bath

To enhance your bath experience, mix 1 teaspoon of sea/Epsom salts and approximately 6-9 drops of Geranium essential oil in a small bowl. Once your bath is filled, pour the mixture into the water and get in. Allow your body to ease into the water and take a moment to inhale the soothing aroma of the oil. Relax and meditate while listening to a guided meditation of your choosing.

Another suggestion would be to imagine Nityaklinna in her customary form or as depicted in Botticelli's 'The Birth of Venus'. I've discovered that this method of visualization often yields deep and meaningful insights.

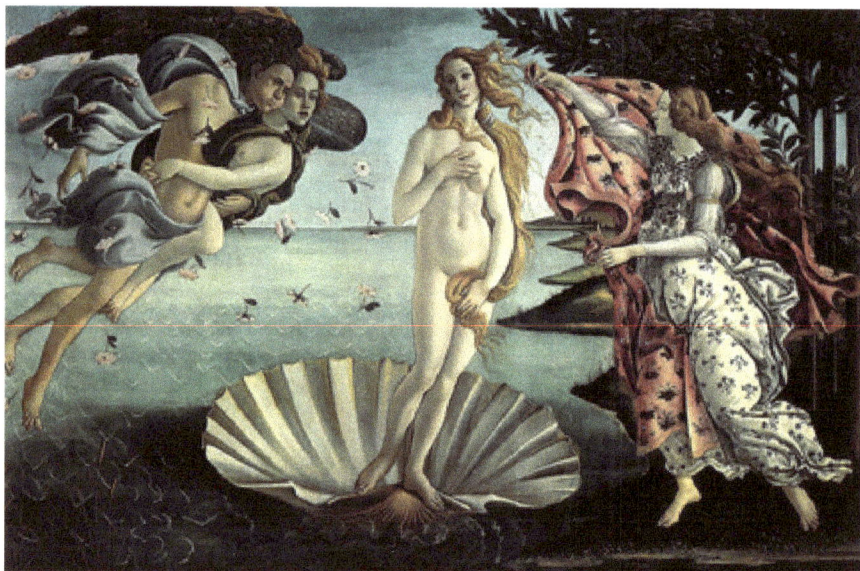

Botticelli's 'The Birth of Venus' Photo courtesy of wiki commons.
wikimedia.org/wiki/File:La,nascita,di,Venere,(Botticelli).jpg)

Like in a dream
I see you
Coming out of the water
Your wet hair is a golden halo
of liquid stars
Pouring over your body
Your soft skin smeared with red sandal paste,
Shimmering Amrita on your thighs
Reflecting rainbows

Onto your temple
A timeless vision of
She,
Who is eternally
Wet with love

4. Waxing Moon
Shivaduti – Duti (The messenger)

On the night of the waxing moon, ideas, thoughts and projects that were conceived on the new moon, are starting to take shape and we begin to see and understand their full potential. The waxing moon signifies growth and transformation, like a messenger, the light half of the moon appears in the night sky, bringing news of what is to come. It reminds us of the perfect balance between light and dark, the realisation that one cannot exist without the other.

On the Kala Mandala, the seventh night is characterized by the influence, inspiration, and playful spirit of Shivaduti.

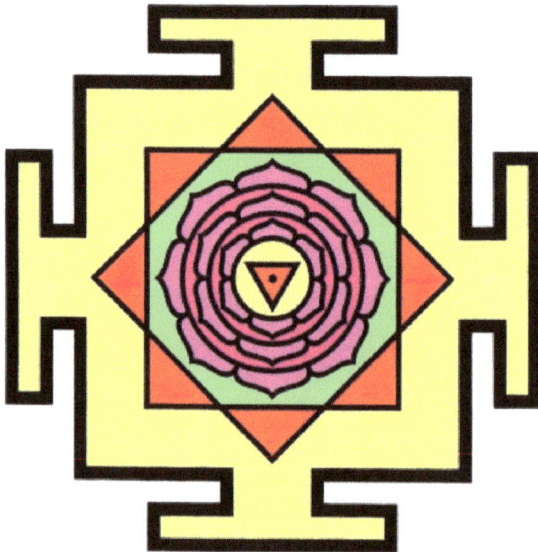

Shivaduti yantra

'She who is full of light and splendour. She who has an aura of light'. 'She for whom Siva is the messenger'

(The Thousand Names of the Divine Mother p.192)

The name Shivaduti signifies a messenger of Shiva and is a significant embodiment of the divine feminine energy, Shakti. She played a crucial role in the battle against the demons Shumbha and Nishumbha, representing the incomparable strength of the Goddess. Shivaduti represents the formidable and mighty manifestation of Shakti that can suppress Adharma - the state of chaos, disharmony, and disorder, and restore equilibrium to the cosmos. *The Tantraraja* (Translation - Mike Magee - shivashakti.com) describes her as being dressed in red, with nine jewels in her crown, surrounded by Rishis singing her praises and having eight arms and three eyes. She looks as bright as the summer sun at midday and smiles sweetly. According to Gregory Peters, "She is sometimes accompanied by a black jackal or may appear with the head of a jackal" (Yogini Magic). This says to me that she is part of untamed nature and by extension the unformed, chaotic part of our world.

As an enthusiastic aromatherapy student, I loved to experiment with essential oil blends. But I'll never forget the wise words of my teacher, Julian Barker, who urged me to take it one step at a time and first experiment with each oil separately before mixing them together. I was given a specific guideline to follow, which involved spending a duration of 1-3 weeks with each oil. As per the instruction, I made it a point to smell the selected essential oil every day and indulge in a therapeutic bath 2-3 times a week. While learning and exploring the benefits of the Rose. I decided to purchase the best quality Rose essential oil that I could afford. Once I had it in my possession, I hurried back home to commence my experiments.

I recall standing in front of the mirror with my eyes shut, attempting to concentrate on the Rose oil's fragrance, urging it to reveal its secrets to me. As I breathed in the lovely scent, it felt like a cool breeze on a hot day swept through my body, gently caressing my inner organs and reenergizing me. As I peered into the centre of the Rose and examined the intricate details of its delicate petals, a mysterious pathway seemed to emerge and transport me into a world of knowledge and understanding. Though it may seem unbelievable, I had a strong sense that I had just connected with the spirit of the plant and its messenger. I had a sudden realization that our sense of smell is incredibly powerful. It can trigger memories and emotions in an instant, taking us on a journey down memory lane or sending us on an emotional rollercoaster ride.

> "Smells are handled by the olfactory bulb, the structure in the front of the brain that sends information to the other areas of the body's central command for further processing. Odours take a direct route to the limbic system, including the amygdala and the hippocampus, the regions related to emotion and memory. The olfactory signals very quickly get to the limbic system." (Coleen Walsh, "What the Nose Knows" – *The Harvard Gazette, Science & Technology*, online journal accessed 27/2/2020)

After a few days of experimenting with my Rose oil, I had a realization that creating a personalized initiatory oil was necessary. This elevated my oil routine to the next level. Each day, I take a few moments to meditate on the oil's fragrance while inhaling its aroma. Then, I applied it to various pulse points behind my ears, temples, and wrists for maximum effect. Certain areas on the body have major arteries that are closer to the skin's surface, called pulse points. By applying essential oils to these areas, they absorb more rapidly compared to other parts of the body. I thoroughly enjoy taking baths, so incorporating three therapeutic baths a week was an easy addition to my routine. I also decided to extend the recommended

15-minute soak time to 30 minutes or more, as I am a Pisces and feel most at home in the water.

The experiment with the Rose essential oil lasted much longer than I anticipated. From what I recall, it lasted around three months before strange things started happening and I had to put an end to it.

For weeks, I felt like I was on top of the world. I was overflowing with insights and ideas that seemed to come to me out of nowhere. Looking back, it almost felt like I was entering into a magical realm filled with synchronicities, spiritual insights, and a sense of euphoria, unlike anything I had ever experienced before. It was as if I was riding the waves of some kind of alchemical process, and I could see crystal clear, almost like I had gained some kind of superpower. Everything I did or said during those weeks just felt right, like I was becoming unstoppable.

Or was I?

One morning, as I was getting ready and applying some Rose oil to my pulse points, something strange caught my eye in the mirror. It was almost like a scene out of a dream or a fantasy film. As I gazed into the mirror, my reflection appeared distorted with delicate Rose leaves twining around my neck and behind my ears. I had Rose petals all over my hair and a huge Rose was looming behind me, almost as if it could engulf me. I spent some time staring at my reflection in the mirror before putting away the Rose oil and splashing my face with cold water. The strange vision I had disappeared. The next day, I talked to my aromatherapy teacher, the late Sheila Brooke, about what happened. She suggested that I avoid using Rose oil in the future. At that point, I was feeling down but I knew it was necessary to let go. Back then, I couldn't comprehend the reason behind it all as I believed that I was on the verge of discovering something amazing. It was only years later, during an ayahuasca ceremony, that I recognized the true value of what I had experienced. It was a precious gift, a brief glimpse into the essence of the Rose, the messenger of the divine mother.

> "...the Rose is the Absolute Self-Sacrifice, the merging of all in the O (negative), the Universal Principle of generation through change (not merely the feminine), and the Universal Light 'khabs'. (Aleister Crowley, *The Confessions* p. 192)

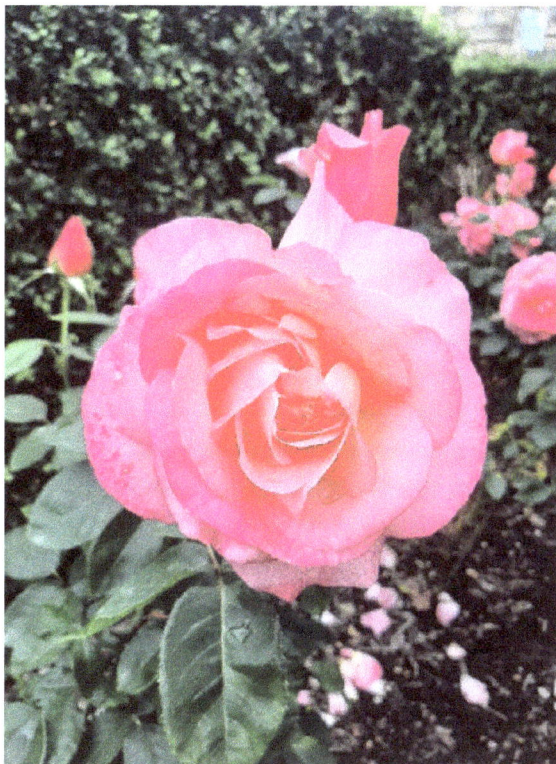

Rose, *Rosa damascena*

(Author's photograph)

Rosa damascena is a type of shrub that can grow up to 2 metres high and has pink, fragrant flowers and grey-green leaves. It is mainly grown in Bulgaria, Turkey, and France and is one of three subspecies that are distilled for their perfume, alongside Rosa gallica and Rosa centifolia.

The Rose has such a beautiful and captivating scent, no wonder it's considered one of the most powerful of healing tools. Its frequency vibrates at 320 MHz, the highest frequency of all living and substantial things that we can experience with our senses. It's amazing to think that something as simple as smelling a Rose can have such a profound effect on our well-being and bring us closer to feelings of love and healing. The

528 Hz Solfeggio Frequency, or 'the love frequency', is thought to resonate at the core of everything, connecting our heart and our spiritual nature to divine harmony. The Solfeggio frequency is believed to affect the conscious and subconscious mind and stimulate healing and promote vitality.

The human body has a vibrational frequency that extends down to the cellular level, the higher the frequency, the better our health. Studies have indicated that a typical healthy body has a frequency range of 62-72 MHz. Therefore, it is understandable that when we come across a Rose, each of our cells is vibrating and opening up, attempting to synchronize with the "love frequency" and luxuriate in the therapeutic splendour of this magnificent flower. The Rose was hailed as the 'queen of flowers' by the ancient Greek poet Sappho, highlighting its delicate aroma and therapeutic benefits that have secured its position in the field of medicine and perfumery.

In comparison to some other essential oil frequencies, you can see clearly why the name 'the queen of flowers' is perfect for our Rose:

Rose   320 MHz
Helichrysum 180 MHz
Frankincense 147 MHz
Lavender   118 MHz
Chamomile   105 MHz
Juniper   98 MHz
Sandalwood   98 MHz

The Rose's high frequency is also said to resonate with the angelic realms, opening a passage for communications with higher beings and the divine. The transformative energies of the waxing moon can be enhanced by the Rose, its sweet and deep scent will indicate and illuminate the cycle ahead of us.

Waxing moon ritual

To prepare the Rose initiation oil for the ritual, gather 1 tablespoon of almond oil and 1-3 drops of Rose essential oil. Combine both ingredients in a small bowl or jar.

Stand in front of a mirror and apply the Rose initiation oil to your pulse points. These include your temples, behind your ears, on your wrists, and under your nose. To enhance the experience, you can warm the oil by rubbing your hands together first. Then, gently massage the oil onto your face as if you were applying facial cream. This will create a luxurious sensation as you feel 'bathed' in the fragrant Rose oil.

Stare at your reflection in the mirror, inhale the scented oil and say:

Goddess of the 7th lunar day,

A special kind of messenger,
Letting your heart know,
A devotee is waiting for you in the special place,
Will you come,
& commune the secrets of existence via
the sweetest scented flower in your lunar garden
As you engage in this simple yet powerful meditation, allow yourself to attune to the highest frequencies. By opening your heart and being honest with yourself as you focus on the Rose, you will gain greater access to communication, insights, and higher knowledge.

* * *

If you don't have any Rose essential oil available, you can try using Rose incense or a fresh Rose flower instead. For the incense, simply light it and allow the aromatic smoke to surround you while you meditate in front of a mirror. If you choose to use a Rose flower, make sure it has a strong fragrance before inhaling its aroma while meditating in front of the mirror.

5. Full Moon
The 16th Kala / Amrita – Lalita

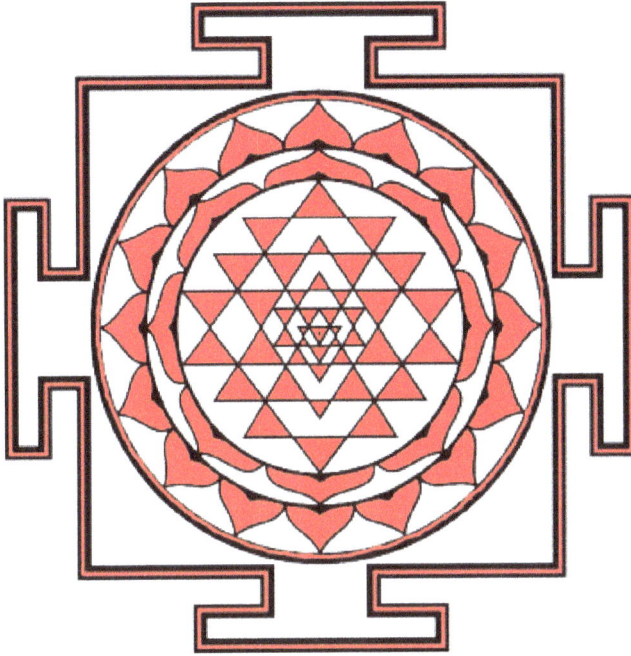

Sri Yantra

"The Shri Chakra is the moon in its fullness, the lotus in full flower, the flow-er which, in the graded phases of its cycle, emanates fourteen rays (one for each day of the fortnight) that culminate in the full circle of the fifteenth."

"From the sixteenth ray or digit of the moon flows "the nectar of supreme excellence". According to the Lalitasahasranama, "the moon shows fifteen phases in its waxing and waning. The sixteenth part, when Time stands still, is when and where Divinity incarnates". Time is Kali, the Goddess Fifteen, and the kala that transcends time is known as the sixteenth digit or ray." (Kenneth Grant, *Aleister Crowley and The Hidden God*, p.26)

Amrita means "immortality" and is often referred to in ancient Indian texts as nectar or ambrosia. It is first mentioned in the Rigveda, where it is considered to be one of the several synonyms for Soma, the drink of the devas. The Sixteenth Kala is associated with Lalita and can be thought of as "outside the circle of time" (Kenneth Grant), she is the 16th Kala in a 15 Kalas sequence. The Sixteenth Kala resonates with the sexual magic elixir. She initiates and awakens the kundalini serpent, its power vibrating with each Kala, reaching its full potential power on the full moon. From the full moon back to the new moon, we experience the manifesting reflective aspect of the kundalini serpent.

Lalita means 'She Who Plays', she is believed to be the representation of the five elements: earth, water, air, fire, and space. Lalita is the embodiment of all creation, manifestation, and dissolution that transcends time. She is the purest form of spirit and pure sattva (truth, balance and peace). She has the power to create and destroy all things by herself.

The Sri Yantra portrays the Goddess in the form of Devi Tripura Sundari — the natural beauty of the three worlds:

1. The world of the Physical Plane, the consciousness of the Physical Plane.

2. The Intermediate Space, Sub-Consciousness of the Prana (breath).

3. The Heaven or Super-Consciousness of the Divine Mind.

It also represents the evolution of the multiverse as a result of the natural Divine Will of the Godhead Aadi Paraa Shakti (the supreme goddess).

The representation of the Goddess's masculine form is depicted by four upward-pointing isosceles triangles, whereas the female embodiment is signified by five downward-pointing triangles. These triangles are encompassed by two concentric circles consisting of 8 and 16 petals, signifying the Lotus of creation and reproductive energy.

The Nymphaea lotus, also known as the white Egyptian lotus, tiger lotus, white lotus or Egyptian water Lily, is a flowering plant of the family Nymphaeaceae and is distributed in various parts of East Africa and Southeast Asia. The white Lotus flower opens after sunset and for 3 nights it blooms for about 16 hours between 8 pm to midday. Once open, it reveals the golden sunset colours of its sunray-like stigma and its white petals symmetry. The striking bloom of the Egyptian water Lily is visible both night and day and symbolises the Night Sun i.e. the Moon, and was considered a symbol of creation and transformation. The Lotus also represents the concept of primordial birth from the cosmic waters of creation.

The colour white is often associated with purity, cleanliness or something new. It also represents a blank canvas — a fresh start. While the petals of the Lotus are white and pure, the plant's roots, are deeply embedded in muddy water, signifying the contrast between light and dark.

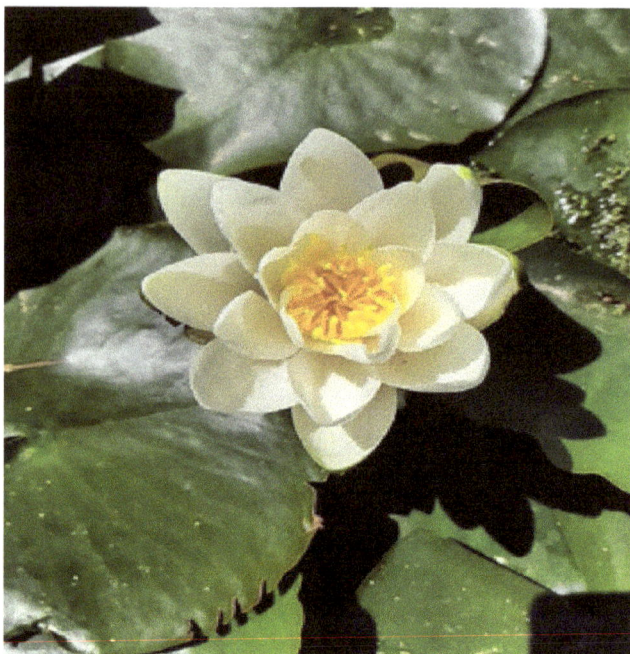

White Lotus, Nymphaea lotus

(Photo by the author)

By connecting with the Sixteenth Kala, we can gain a deeper understanding of the complete cycle of the Kalas. I find that the best methods to resonate with the Kalas are meditation, visualisation and the use of essential oils. My personal favourite is a combination of all three. When we take a ritual bath, we can establish a holy atmosphere where our physical and mental states can align with the moon's essence and its gravitational influence over us.

During the full moon, Shakti has reached the peak of her cycle and is now flourishing, ready to bring forth a fresh wave of Kalas. Her cup is overflowing with the sacred nectar, known as Soma. At this moment, she is Lalita and Amrita. The waxing moon has completed its cycle and for a brief moment, time seems to pause, granting us the chance to experience both the past and the future. The radiance of Lalita's playground has shone upon us, and the deeds we undertook during the new moon have become deeply ingrained in our minds and souls. Luna, heavily pregnant with ideas and dreams, is ready to give birth to her most extraordinary magic; the timeless cycle of birth and death.

Like the white Lotus, the intense scent of Jasmine can also affect our emotions by producing feelings of optimism, confidence and euphoria; on the spiritual level, it promotes creativity, intuition, and insights. It also stimulates original ideas and dreams. I find that Jasmine is the perfect oil for a "scentual" evocation of the Sixteenth Kala, helping us give birth and release the new thoughts and concepts we have planted on the new moon and get charged again with her illuminating light.

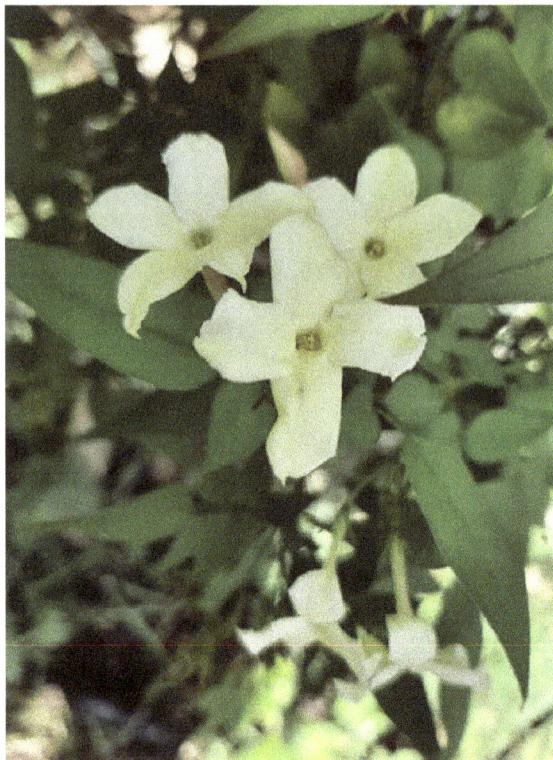

Jasmine, Jasminum officinale

(Photo by the author)

Jasmine is an evergreen shrub that can grow up to ten metres high. It has delicate star-shaped white flowers and bright green leaves. Jasmine flowers are intensely sweet and have an exquisite and deep aroma. Jasmine is native to China, northern India and West Asia. Jasmine essential oil can be used for sensitive skin, muscular spasms, labour pains, nervous exhaustion and stress-related conditions.

Jasmine essential oil is one of the must-have oils in the doula working kit. It is one of the most valued oils during childbirth as it can help relieve pain, strengthen contractions and disperse fears, bringing love and euphoria to the birth of a new life. Jasmine is also considered an aphrodisiac and sexual tonic.

During my time as a doula, I recall a particular client who was adamant about using only Jasmine oil during her labour. She explained that other oils in my kit, such as Clary Sage, Rose, and Lavender (to name a few) made her feel sick. This woman was a strong-willed individual, and once she made up her mind, it was difficult to sway her. However, upon arriving at the delivery room, she remained tense and was quite demanding towards me, the midwife, the nurse and her husband. All of us were aware that her attitude had to be shifted if we were expecting a trouble-free delivery. As such, I used a bit of pure Jasmine essential oil on a tissue and requested her to inhale deeply. Concurrently, I began rubbing her feet and after some time she asked me to knead her lower back while she was still attempting to smell the scented tissue. It didn't take long for the atmosphere in the delivery room to change and we collaborated without a word in an aromatic symphony. Finally, my client allowed herself to let go and surrendered herself to the birthing process and the very capable hands of the midwife. She seemed to be in an ecstatic trance, in a state of bliss. All of us in the room were experiencing something which I can only describe as a spiritual high and with one mighty contraction, she delivered the most beautiful healthy baby, and all of us, midwife and nurse included, burst into tears.

My time as a doula has seen many memorable moments, and this birth was certainly one of them. Whether it was down to the soothing effects of Jasmine oil or the powerful Oxytocin - often referred to as the "hormone of love" - its impact will stay with me forever. When I reunited with the parents a few days after, I inquired about their experience. Her answer said it all "We decided to name the baby Jasmine".

The Sixteenth Kala bath ritual

Gather 1 tablespoon of Epsom or sea salt, and if you prefer, substitute it for powdered milk. In a small bowl or jar, mix the salts (or powder) with 2-3 drops of Jasmine essential oil.

When your bath is full, add the blend to it and swirl your hand in a figure of eight. Focus on your intentions and prayers, then relax into the water with closed eyes. Inhale the aroma of the oil while listening to a guided meditation of your preference.

Full moon meditations:

> Here is the supreme sixteenth Kala of the moon.
>
> She is pure and resembles the young sun.
>
> She is as thin as the hundredth part of fibre in the stalk of a lotus.
>
> She is lustrous and soft like ten million lightning flashes and is down-turned.
>
> From her, whose source is the Brahman, flows copiously the continuous stream of nectar. (Arthur Avalon, *The Serpent Power*, Verse 46)
>
> She, the Primordial Sakti who excels all and who, in Her own true nature, is eternal, limitless Bliss is the seed of all the moving and motionless things which are to be, and is the Pure Mirror in which Siva, the Absolute, Experience Himself. (*Ama Kala Vilasa Verse*)

I suggest that you pre-record the Khonsu Invocation and then play it while taking a bath for an enhanced experience. After that, I recommend 'Drawing Down the Moon' outside as a conclusion to your ritual.

Khonsu invocation

I am the one who appears shining and endures

My body grows old when I delay

For I am the serpent that came forth from the Nun,

I am the proud Ethiopian,

I am rearing serpent of real gold,

There is honey on my lips;

That which I shall say cometh to pass.

I am Anubis, the baby creature;

I am Isis and I will bind him,

I am Osiris the drowned who is bound.

Save me from every danger

Protect me, heal me, give me love, praise and reverence

Into my cup here today.

Come to me, Isis, mistress of magic,

the great sorceress of all the gods.

Horus is before me, Nephthys as my diadem...

Send the mighty lion sons of Mihos

Send the souls of god,

The souls of man,

The souls of the Underworld,

The souls of the horizon,

The spirits, the dead,

Come into my cup and tell me the truth today

Concerning that after which I am inquiring:

I summon all your souls and forms to the mouth

Of my vessel;

Let them talk with their mouths,

Let them speak with their lips,

Let them say about that which I ask

Come into me,

South, North, West, East,

Every breeze of Amenti, for I am the fury of all these gods,

Whose names I have uttered here today,

Rouse them for me,

The drowned, the dead; let your soul

and your form live for me

Even the fury of Apophis and her daughters I summon

from their places of punishment,

Let him make me answer to every word [about]

which I am asking here today in truth without

falsehood therein. Hasten,

Quickly!

When outside and bathing in the moonlight, stretch your arms above your head and draw down the moon into you.

Drawing Down the Moon:

I draw down the bright blue Moon from the sky

though brazen cymbals crash and thunder

to keep her in her place;

even the chariot of the Sun,

my grandfather grows pale at my song,

and I drain the colour from the dawn for my potions.

* * *

When a bath is not an option, you can inhale the oil while listening to the mantra/meditation. When Jasmine oil is not available, an alternative is to burn Jasmine incense. After completing your mantra, it is customary to thank the energy/spirit and put the bottle away. In the case that you are using incense, allow it to burn until it has finished.

Another oil that I find resonates perfectly with the Sixteenth Kala is the

Opoponax oil (See Baphomet invocation perfume oil) which corresponds with the qualities of the Kala of the full moon. The essences of both the oil and the Kala, can give us clarity and insights into the cycle ahead and restore balance and harmony in our body and mind.

When our minds and hearts are resonating with the oil and the Kala, we can experience the most magical and transforming journey. Opoponax oil, like the Sixteenth Kala, protects us from negativity and promotes intuition and magical vision.

6. Kali

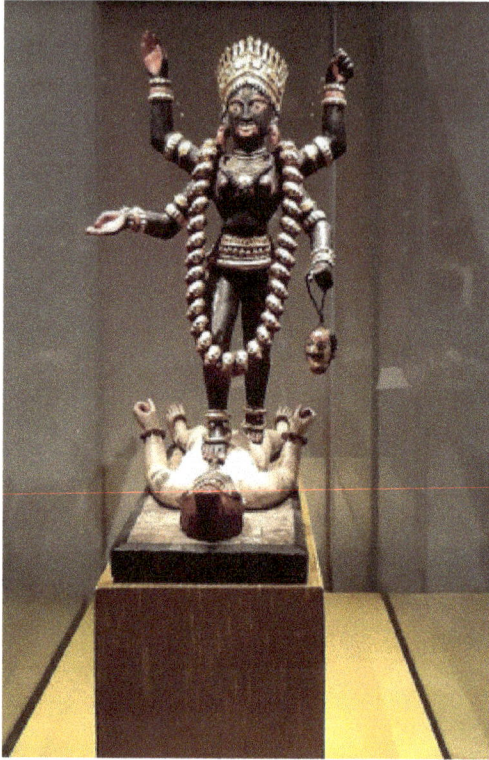

"I am Great Nature, consciousness, bliss, the quintessence, devotedly praised. Where I am, there are no Brahama, Hara, Sambhu or other devas, nor is there creation, maintenance or dissolution. Where I am, there is no attachment, happiness, sadness, liberation, goodness, faith, atheism, guru or disciple" (*Kali Magic*, Mike Magee)

Kali is the 15th Kala and the last Kala on the Shakti/light sequence, but also the first Kala on the dark/Kali sequence.

She represents the full moon and the initiation of the dark cycle of the moon phase. While Lalita represents the embodiment of all creation, manifestation, and dissolution that transcends time, Kali is Time itself and the manifestation of the eternal moment. You might be wondering how Lalita can be both creation itself and the full moon after what was said in the last chapter. Lalita is beyond our comprehension of time and space and can only manifest when the "Time is right." Through devotion and total surrender to the Goddess Kali, one realises the illusion of time and witnesses Lalita's magical manifestation during a full moon. The moon cycle consists of two different sequences: the 'light' sequence of Shakti (waxing moon) and the 'dark or Kali' sequence (waning moon). Each sequence has 15 Kalas, each representing a phase of the moon for every day of the month.

Miryamdevi's poem describes this well:

For 15 days and nights,
We are shining bright
Happy
Dancing
Kissing
Telling little love stories
to each other
The stories of Kameshvari and her
ankle bracelet
Duti The impossible girl messenger
and ChitraMalini-
The bright one
The full one
The one who initiates her twin sister-
Kali
Tonight is the 15th night of

sweet love
Long kisses
Passion and desires
I am Shakti
The Lady of desire
Messenger of love
Bright garland
The Kiss of life
I am Shakti
My eyes shine like
Two bright suns
but if you look closely

You will see
Two black suns rising inside
I am Kali
I am the dark one
You can only see me
when the moon is full.
I am Kali

On the 15th night, Kali Kala night, Time is transcended and we are experiencing the Eternal Moment. Kali's Time is divided into 30 Kalas and each one of them teaches us how to experience the moment to its fullest. When Time manifests itself during a full moon, we are granted magical boons and a glimpse into Lalita's illuminating bright glow. Lalita embodies all creation, manifestation, and dissolution that transcends Time into one existing moment — the Eternal moment, Kali.

The only Time is Now, and Now is the moment.

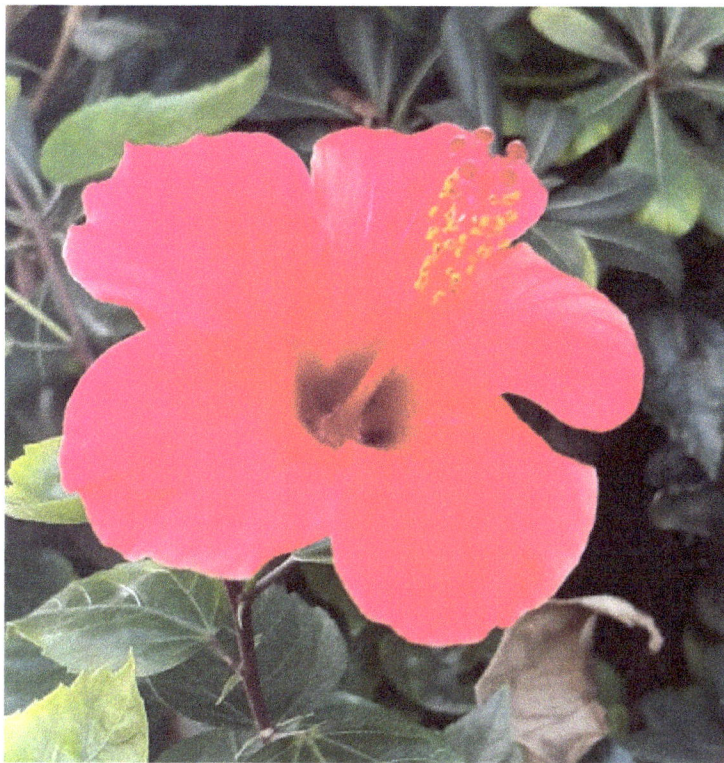

Hibiscus, *Rosa sinensis*

(Photo by the author)

The vivid red of the Hibiscus serves as a reminder of Kali's primordial energy, its specific significance in Hindu mythology rooted in her embodiment of Shakti - cosmic energy and mother of all living forms. Representing empowerment and destruction, the Hibiscus captures her unbridled power and strong presence. The red Hibiscus has immense spiritual connotations in Hinduism; representing Kali's grace and divine intervention, it conveys the protection of devotees and negates all negative energies. This flower acts as an offering to the Goddess, a demonstration of the surrender of desires and ego, for her protection.

Ambrette Seed oil is a valuable essential oil that is extracted from the fully ripened seeds of a type of Hibiscus plant. This evergreen aromatic shrub, which belongs to the Malvaceae family, can grow up to 1.5 metres high and produces large single flowers. The kidney-shaped seeds have a sweet, woody, slightly herbaceous, flowery heavy fragrance that is similar to that of musk. This popular oil is native to India and is also known as Mushkdana. It is widely cultivated in various parts of the world, including the West Indies, China, Indonesia, Africa, and Egypt.

When I first smelled Ambrette seed oil, I wasn't taken by its scent at all as it was too woody and slightly sharp, which was nothing I had expected for a sacred and spiritual flower fragrance to be. However, I remembered that some descriptions of this essential oil said that the aroma only becomes more pleasant with time - mellowing into a heady and sweet floral-musky concoction reminiscent of wine or brandy, I reconsidered my opinion. I decided to make a dilution of the oil and see what would happen. I couldn't help but open the bottle a few weeks after diluting it by 5%. To my surprise, the aroma had evolved into something more delightful; gone was its sharp woody scent and in its place was a floral sweetness with a distinct musky aroma. Having studied the Goddess Kali for many years, it was devotion and total surrender that led me to appreciate her unfolding like a flower and scentual essence. There is something about Ambrette Seed oil that compels the senses and awakens desire, recognised to affect the base chakra and Kundalini snake - both integral elements in tantric practices.

> "According to the *Kaulajnananirnaya*, offering flowers with no perfume does not please the goddess." (Magee 2022)

After I first read the quote, I knew that I would offer perfume oil to Kali, incorporating the most aromatic blooms. Therefore, Mimosa was the next essential oil to go in the bottle (see information in the following chapter).

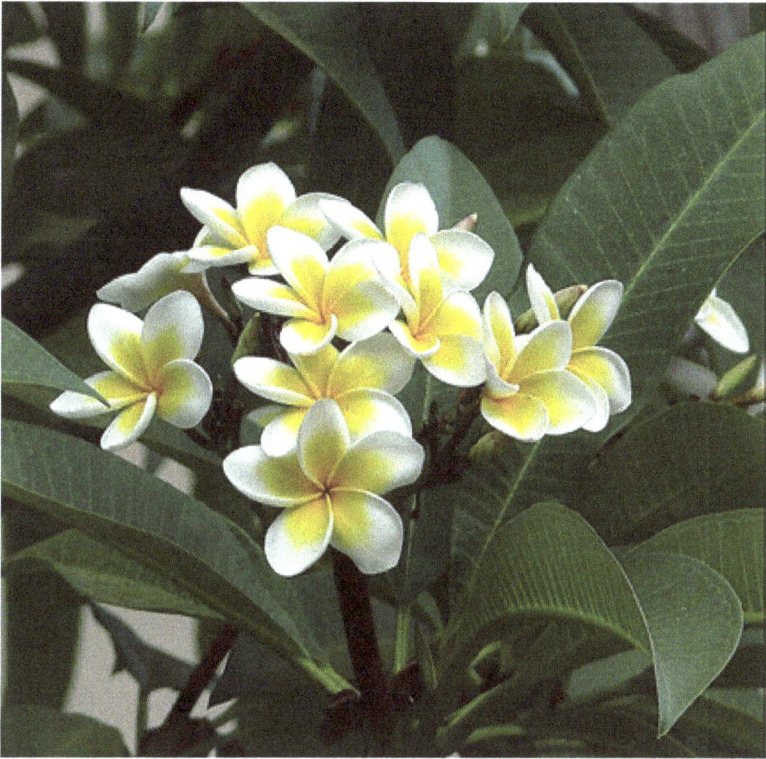

Frangipani, *Plumeria alba*

(Photo courtesy of wiki commons.
wikimedia.org/wiki/File:Plumeria-0006-Zachi-Evenor.jpg)

Plumeria is a genus of flowering plants that belong to the family Apocynaceae and the subfamily Rauvolfioideae. The trees can grow up to 5 metres with their leaves at the tips of their branches. They flower from early summer to fall and their blossoms grow in clusters on the ends of the stems. The flowers are highly fragrant, especially at night and are made of tubular corolla that split into five rounded and waxy petals that overlap each other. They are also known as Frangipani. The flowers come in many colours including pink, red, white and yellow, orange, or pastel. Plumeria varieties are native to Mexico, Central America, Brazil and the Caribbean. They grow widely throughout the Far East, India and many tropical and warm parts of the world.

The plant was named after a 16th-century marquess from the Frangipani family, Muzio Frangipane. Other names for these species vary depending on region and type, but Frangipani remains a popular name for them. It is said that Muzio created a fragrant perfume with the scent of Plumeria which may explain why this genus is called by his surname. Frangipani has a sweet and fresh aroma that is unique and exotic. It has heady and intoxicating vibes and is an alluring aroma that is invigorating, euphoric and a stimulating aphrodisiac for the body and mind. Its unusual fragrance and uplifting and soothing characteristics, make Frangipani essential oil one of the most attractive and attention-grabbing scents that has earned its place in the use of the high-class perfumery.

In India, Plumeria is known as the Tree of Life. It is believed that a branch cut from the tree will continue to blossom as if representing our soul's infinite connection to the Divine. Frangipani was a favourite flower of Lord Krishna. In the Tantrik tradition, Krishna is often identified with Kali. In the Todala Tantra, each of the ten Mahavidyas, forms of the supreme Goddess, has her own male counterpart and here Krishna is said to be the spouse of Kali. There are many images of Krishna in India which show him as black. Kali and Krishna form a divine unity. The Tantrik texts of Bengal give much more mention of this inseparable form. In the *Tantrarajatantra*'s 4th chapter that glorifies Lalita, it is said that she enchanted men and to enchant women, Lalita took the form of Krishna. The Bengali text of Kalivilasa Tantra mentions Krishna as the son of Devi who was golden and turned black when he was excited by passion. During the full moon, it is not uncommon to experience heightened magical manifestations and illusions. As we learned earlier in this chapter, Lalita can only manifest through Kali, who is in divine unity with Krishna. This amplifies the spiritual energy and mystical experiences we may encounter during this time. Kali is the embodiment of time, possessing the power to both create and destroy all that exists. The pyre signifies her essence, a great fire that burns at the end of time. It is said to be located at the centre of the spine, generating immense joy and consuming all internal illusions during the ecstasy of enlightenment. This is also the fire that awakens the female serpent, Kundalini.

It is said that Kundalini resides at the bottom of the spine nesting amidst the three principal Nadis or channels. According to traditional Indian medicine and spiritual theory, the Nadis are the channels through which the prana energy of the physical body, subtle body and causal body flows (Prana can be translated from Sanskrit as life force, vital energy, breath of life, spiritual energy, or the vital principle). The three principal Nadis are Ida, Pingala, and Sushumna. Ida lies to the left of the spine, whereas Pingala is to the right. Sushumna runs along the spinal cord in the centre. When the channels are unblocked through Yoga and Pranayama, breathing exercises, the Kundalini energy uncoils and rises up Sushumna from the base of the spine.

The fire at the end of time is the great fire of creation. When our Nadis are clear of obstacles and the Prana is flowing free, Kundalini will start to uncoil and move upward in a spiral dance of creation. The latter is like the double helix of DNA which is essentially a three-dimensional spiral. The double -stranded molecule could both produce exact copies of itself and carry genetic instructions. The double helix serves as a small-scale, personal representation of how cells are created, providing the necessary information to form each person's unique genetic code. On the other hand, Kundalini represents a larger-scale picture of creation, encompassing universal and cosmological events and serving as the original code of the Goddess.

Kali is described as the divine Shakti embodying both the constructive and destructive forces of nature, She is the goddess who represents both life-giving and death-bringing powers. Kali is often depicted draped only in the veil of the cosmos, with her blue-black nakedness signifying the eternal void of non-existence, a state free from any kind of illusion or differentiation. She is regarded as the epitome of pure and fundamental reality, the underlying structure of all things, an unfathomable void that is formless and full of potential.

The deities Vishnu, Krishna, and Shiva are also often portrayed with a skin tone that is blue or dusky. This colour is representative of the boundless and incomprehensible and reminds us that what we perceive as these divine figures is actually the omnipresent reality. By giving form to the formless Brahman (God), our minds are aided in understanding through the colour blue. Kali embodies the entirety of the physical world. She encompasses all the emotions and experiences that come with life. She fills the roles of brother, father, sister, mother, lover, and friend, but also embodies darker personas such as fiend, monster, beast, and brute. The sun and the ocean, the grass and the dew, all are a part of her essence. Our sense of accomplishment and satisfaction is tied to her, as is our sense of discovery and wonder. She is the epitome of a full and seductive but fearsome earth mother, always ready to offer something new and exciting.

According to Kenneth Grant, "The dark fortnight comprised the period from full to new moon". Even though Kali's sequence is considered the dark sequence, from my own personal experience I can say that each one of the Kalas on the darker side of the moon, brings a vast illumination into the process of the waning moon and its descent into darkness. During this time, our minds will adapt to the dark blue colour of the night sky and will have a chance to experience the boundless, eternal void full of potential that is the Goddess.

I have crafted Kali's Perfume oil blend as an offering to Devi, the instigator of Kali Magick. Every breath of its scent transports me to an experience of pure thankfulness and oneness with the divine. The aroma of the Goddess draws us into a feeling of permanence, encouraging us to fully embrace the present moment and assume it will remain eternal.

7. Kulla & Kurukulla
Kulla "The Ancestral"

"She who is the deity in the kulas, the essence of the universe and the essence of knowledge" (Sri Lalita Sahsranama, *The Thousand Names of the Divine Mother*)

Kulla is aroused on the third-day after the full moon, and her name represents the world and its knowledge, suggesting she's deeply connected to the cosmos. Furthermore, Kula can mean "home," implying that her energy does inhabit a particular area. Still basking in the moon's light, Kulla indicates that the waning moon is in progress and reminds us of the eternal cycle of birth and death. She teaches us the secrets of transformations and gives us a glimpse into the

"Ein Sof – אֵין סוֹף ", helping us to understand the concepts of 'Eternal', 'All is one' and 'The Void'. Kula allows us to attain a state in which we are oblivious to the concept of time, position, movement, origin and consequence.

Kula marks the gate in the lunar cycle, through which we can access our ancestors. Any supplications to them will be powerfully welcomed on this day. Personally, I always try to spend some time tending the forebears' altar: cleansing it, dusting it off and adding fresh flowers and offerings. A particular pleasure I have is drying various blooms on this altar, finding that doing so brings out a luminous vibrancy in their hues beyond what I get elsewhere in the house.

For all sorts of reasons, some of us will find it difficult to respect or pay homage to ancestors from our own bloodline. I believe that our ancestors can be anyone that influenced us and has shaped the way we think and do things. Their iconic memory represents all of those who came before us on the path we choose to take. You may find that it includes anyone from a beloved family member to a famous figure such as a Hollywood starlet, musician, author or thinker from the past. The important thing is that you feel a deep connection to their essence and carry their legacy within your heart and actions.

Whichever ancestors you are honouring, do it with all the respect and understanding of their traditions and history. After discovering your ancestry, it is time to set your ancestral altar accordingly. Anything that will remind you of your ancestors can be placed on the altar. I also like to put a candle, incense and a cup of water that represent the Source of life itself. In some traditions, the ancestor's favourite food or drink, perfume and tobacco will also be placed on the altar as an offering. Follow your heart and intuition when creating an altar. Esthetically and emotionally, the altar should please and move you, after all, it is your focal point in time and space to take a break from the everyday rat run and connect with the spirit of your ancestors.

Spikenard resonates with the essence of Kula, the ancestor.

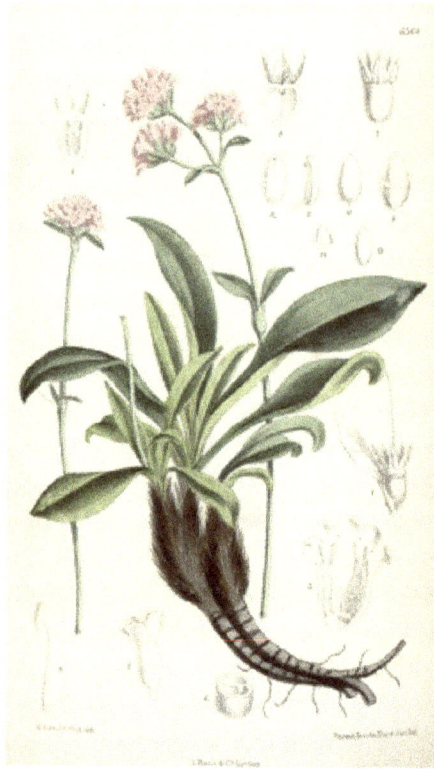

Spikenard, Nardostachys jatamansi

(Photo courtesy of wiki commons.wikimedia.org/wiki/
File:Nardostachys,grandiflora.jpg)

Spikenard, known also as Nard or Jatamansi, is a small, delicate herb with an aromatic rhizome, of the botanical family of Valerianaceae. It is native to the mountain areas of north India, China and Japan. The essential oil is extracted by steam distillation from the dried and crushed rhizomes and roots.

One of the first fragrances to be utilized by ancient civilizations along the incense trade route from India to the Middle East was Spikenard. Due to its perceived sacredness and high cost, it was deemed a precious commodity. Traditional medicine, perfumery, and religious ceremonies all made use of this revered plant by various cultures such as Hindus,

Hebrews, Egyptians, Greeks and Romans. The popularity of spikenard is evident in its inclusion in multiple biblical passages mentioned in the Song of Solomon.

> Song 1:12 While the king sits at his table, my spikenard forth the smell thereof.

> Song 4:13 Your plants are an orchard of pomegranates, with pleasant fruits; camphire, with spikenard,

> Song 4:14 Spikenard and saffron; calamus and cinnamon, with all trees of frankincense; myrrh and aloes, with all the chief spices

The therapeutic powers of spikenard are numerous, including anti-inflammatory, antipyretic, bactericidal and fungicidal qualities, in addition to its ability to act as a laxative, sedative and tonic. With knowledge of these healing benefits, it is easy to understand why Mary Magdalene may have chosen it for use with Jesus. Nardostachys jatamansi, otherwise known as Spikenard, is believed to embody a spiritual essence. The Nepalese name Jatamansi, meaning 'spirit', gives us an insight into the possible spiritual applications of this herb.

Mary Magdalene

The first time Spikenard is mentioned in the New Testament is Mark 14:3

> "And being in Bethany in the house of Simon the leper, as he sat at meat, there came a woman having an alabaster box of ointment of spikenard very precious; and she brake the box, and poured it on his head."

Mary Magdalene was one of Jesus's disciples and her symbolic act of pouring the oil on his head demonstrated her devotion to him and the recognition of his ancestry and heritage as the Holy King. Oil was used to anoint the kings of the house of David and the high priests of Israel, it served to sanctify them and set them apart as God's chosen rulers. Oil was also utilized for various purposes such as healing, demonstrating honour towards someone, and sanctifying individuals or objects.

Mary Magdalene's choice of Spikenard was not arbitrary, as mentioned above, Spikenard was used in many religious rites by many civilizations. It has been one of the major oils for spiritual transition and resonates with the energy of death (See Felicity Warner, *Sacred Oils*). Spikenard oil, an invaluable aid in aiding spiritual transformation, can support the mind and body of the terminally ill as they accept their fate. It is notable that its healing and transcendental properties were not widely known; moreover, it was considered an extravagant item due to its cost.

> "…there came a woman having an alabaster box of ointment of spikenard very precious; …"(Mark 14:3)

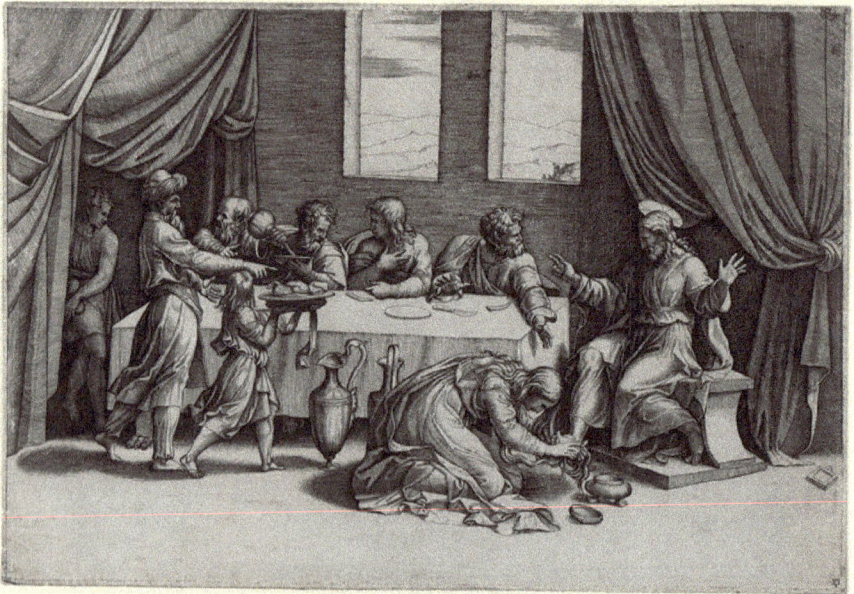

Christ at the table of Simon the Pharisee, Mary Magdalene washing his feet with her hair print, Marcantonio Raimondi, circa 1520–25. (courtesy of wikimedia.org)

The aforementioned details indicate that Mary Magdalene, a prosperous woman with expertise in healing and herbalism, had a strong bond with Jesus. Being one of his disciples, she observed his spiritual metamorphosis. As an adept healer with knowledge of energies and plants, she was perceptive to the changes occurring in his physical body and mind during this transition. Therefore, she opted for Spikenard to aid him in achieving spiritual ascension.

The second time Spikenard is mentioned is in John 12:3

> "Then took Mary a pound of ointment of spikenard, very costly, and anointed the feet of Jesus, and wiped his feet with her hair: and the house was filled with the odour of the ointment."

The verse starts by telling us that Mary took the expensive oil and anointed Jesus's feet with it. In the Hindu Vedas, the feet are referred to as the "organs of action." The period between the new moon – Kameswari and the waxing moon can be thought of as the first steps out of darkness towards the light. By anointing Jesus' feet, Mary gives us another clue about her beliefs and devotion to Jesus and her recognition and acknowledgement of his spiritual transition. We must bear in mind that foot-washing began as a show of hospitality in Middle Eastern households, where servants or the host's wife would perform this service for visiting guests since they typically wore sandals and had to traverse roads filled with dust. Mary's washing of Jesus' feet may imply a close, personal connection between the two. The feet are associated with the elements of fire. The primaeval vital force spark with each beginning of every movement and initiates the first step into the unknown. According to Ayurveda, all energy channels or meridians (Nadis), begin in the scalp and end in the soles of the feet. Mary used her hair to wipe the oil over Jesus's feet, this also might suggest a strong spiritual connection and intimate bond between Mary and Jesus.

The mention of hair symbolizes the manifestation of change and freedom. By wiping Jesus's feet with her hair, Mary is forming an actual physical bond between them, which initiates the energy cycle that flows from her to Jesus and vice versa. By doing so she gives us another clue about their strong connection and the approaching change. Hair can also signify strength and with the act of wiping the feet with her hair, we can assume that there is an exchange of power flowing from Mary to support and strengthen his first step toward spiritual ascension.

Kula teaches us the secrets of transformations and helps us to understand the concepts of eternity. Connecting with our ancestors, we get a sense of the eternal. Through the initiatory properties of Spikenard, we can deepen our links and connect to different time zones and learn how to welcome the highest spiritual transformation, the ascendance to the higher consciousness of the high priest or a king.

Kurukulla - "The Tribal"
"She who is the cause of Wisdom"

Following the night of the full moon, no trace of Shakti's energizing light can be seen nor any remnant of Lalita's ecstatic ambrosia. With the emergence of Kali, Devourer of Time, this ethereal moment outside the circle of time has gone. If Lalita is the essence of all creation and manifestation, Kali is the essence of all that is Not. She is the dark emptiness of the void, the place where nothing is, but everything is possible. She is the head of the Ouroboros serpent devouring its tail.

Each day of the waning moon is represented by one of her Kala essences, teaching us the magick of the shadows. Still basking in her illuminating light, Kapalini, Skull-Girl, teaches us the importance of being in our bodies and not so much in our heads, acknowledging and focusing our intellect on our physical needs. After all, to maintain our spiritual and magical journey, we need to feed and hydrate our bodies and make sure it is adequately rested and vacated. Kula teaches us the essence of the universe and of knowledge, and the wisdom of our ancestors. These ancestral links and lineages are guiding us, and connecting us back to them through spiritual, fellowship, brotherhood, sorority and or blood. Kapalini and Kula's teachings are the essences of the knowledge of the spiritual body and physiological wisdom – the secrets of the body and blood.

Kurukulla, is the enchantress, the sorceress of dark magic. Kurukulla is "the cause of wisdom" and she uses her magnetizing powers to bring conditions favourable to the path to Enlightenment.

> "She has lustrous crimson skin, and often appears draped in flames that caress her body. Her entire countenance is dynamic energy. She is the Queen of Sorcery and Mistress of Dark Magic. She may be holding a bow and arrow made of crystalline flowers of light. She may also be armed with a trident, with a naga coiled about it. She reaches out with her left hand holding a kapala (large cup made from the cranium of a human skull). In the cup is nectar in the form of luminescent blood, which she may offer to you." (*Yogini Magic* by Gregory Peters)

Kurukulla is depicted as beautiful, voluptuous and seductive. She uses her power to attract, magnetize and mesmerise, to lead us on to the path of transformation and enlightenment. Kurukullas's magic works on the deeper levels of our subconscious mind. By visualising ourselves as one with Her, and connecting to Her divine essence, we begin to realise our own internal beauty.

"She may also be armed with a trident"

The Trishula/trident is a weapon used by both Shiva and Durga. Its three points represent various trinities such as creation, maintenance, and destruction. Past, present, future, and the three gunas (energetic forces that weave together to form the universe and everything in it. Tamas/ stability, Rajas/activity, and Sattva/consciousness).

The Trishula is said to destroy the illusion of the three worlds: the physical world, the forefathers or ancestral world and the world of the mind. Kurukulla initiates within us the powers of the Trishula, the divine weapon of enlightenment and the deeper connection we have with her, our minds will tap into Kurukulla's magic and will gain insight into the true nature of reality.

Magical processes will always involve major transformations. When we engage with Kurukulla's magic, big changes will occur within our mindset which will influence our character and personality. Magnetizing, sensuality and charisma are the nature of Kurukulla magic. Only those who are willing to step into the shadows and accept to drink the red luminescent blood from her kapala will transform and change.

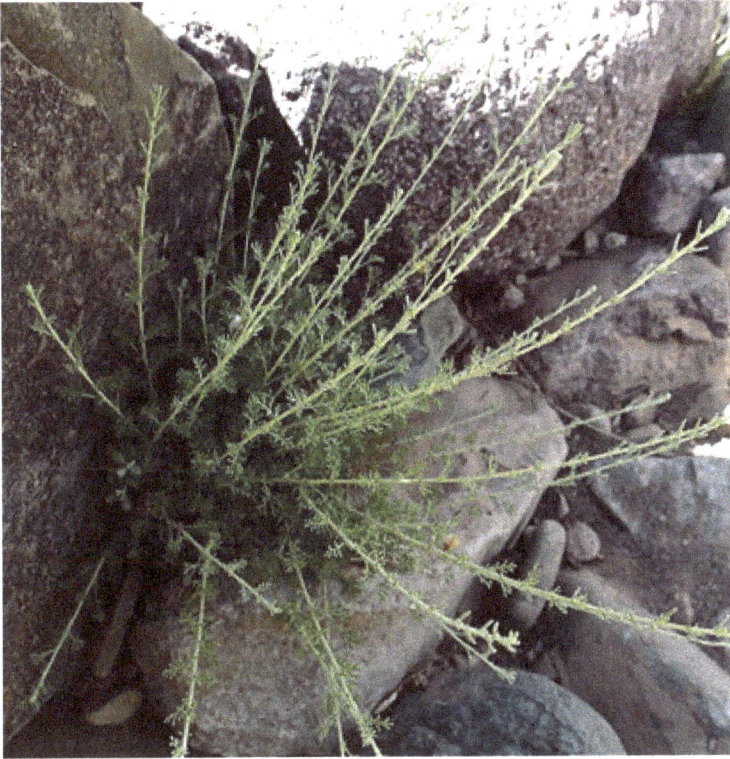

White Wormwood, Artemisia herba-alba

(Photo courtesy of wiki commons.wikimedia.org/wiki/
File:Artemisa,herba,alba,floratrek2013.jpg)

Artemisia herba-alba, the white wormwood, is a small perennial shrub with pale yellow flowers, in the genus Artemisia. It grows commonly on the dryland and prairie of the Mediterranean regions in Northern Africa, the Arabian Peninsula and Southwestern Europe. Wormwood Essential Oil is extracted by steam distillation. The plant exists as various chemotypes and the composition of the oil may vary widely. The specific oil I used here is Moroccan (Marrakesh-type) which has a light herbaceous odour characteristic of thujone.

Essential oils can be classified in several ways and knowing the chemical composition of an oil is a good indication of its therapeutic or possible hazardous effect. Most if not all of the Artemisia species contain a ketone called Thujone.

Organic chemistry examines the structure, properties, and reactions of organic materials which contain carbon atoms. This could range from hydrocarbons (only carbon and hydrogen) to compounds with elements, like nitrogen, oxygen, or hydrogen, included. In short, it is the chemistry found in all living beings. Some of the most common toxic constituents are ketones, such as the thujone found in mugwort, tansy, sage and wormwood. Ketones are generally considered to ease congestion and aid the flow of mucus and they are often found in plants which are used for upper respiratory complaints.

Thujone is a terpene ketone, derived from plants, with volatile properties. In Europe, its use in food and beverages and other consumable products is tightly controlled by the European Parliament and Council and the European Medicines Agency.

Thujone influences the transmission of gamma-aminobutyric acid (GABA) by acting as a competitive antagonist. Its effects, though sometimes stimulating and mood-enhancing at low doses, can be convulsant in certain cases. Furthermore, it is employed in the fragrance industry in many essential oils.

Caution: Wormwood essential oil is for external use only, also, avoid it when pregnant!

Wormwood has a long history of use, with the earliest reference to its existence at least 2,200 years ago. The Huangdi Neijing (The Yellow Emperor's Inner Classic), the earliest written record of Chinese medicine, provides evidence of this from the 3rd century BCE. It is likely that people viewed Wormwood as a magical herb prior to that era.

Wormwood's bitter-green, sharp, fresh top-note fragrance is said to boost psychic skills. Its botanical name derives from the Greek goddess, Artemis and it is sacred also to Lilith. It belongs to the family of Asteraceae, a group consisting of 180 species. It has a strong connection with the spirit world and can be used in rituals performed with or for those that are dying, to ease their transition and enable them to let go. Wormwood is closely related to Mugwort and is extremely powerful when used together for protection and to ward off evil spirits.

As a key ingredient of the Black Magick perfume oil, Wormwood will raise you to a higher level of psychic awareness and will aid in divination and clairvoyance. It is also used in spells for binding, exorcism, protection and powerful aid for evocation, divination, scrying, and prophecy. According to legend, burning the plant in a cemetery will summon the spirits of the departed and if planted around the garden, it will keep pests and snakes away and can be used for boundary magick. Wormwood is thought to have grown from the serpent's path as it left the Garden of Eden.

The potent, captivating power of Kurukulla, the Black Magic sorceress, is contained in the intense bitterness and acetone-like aroma of Wormwood. As the trishula pierces through the delusions of the three worlds, its distinctive freshness will help you unlock your inner sight; merely inhaling its fragrance will make you an acolyte of the 'Tribal One', ready to take on whatever shadows may come. This will then allow for a direct connection to "She that is the source of wisdom".

The ingredients of the Black Magic Perfume Oil signify the luminescent blood in Kurukulla's kapala, the nectar of transformation and change.

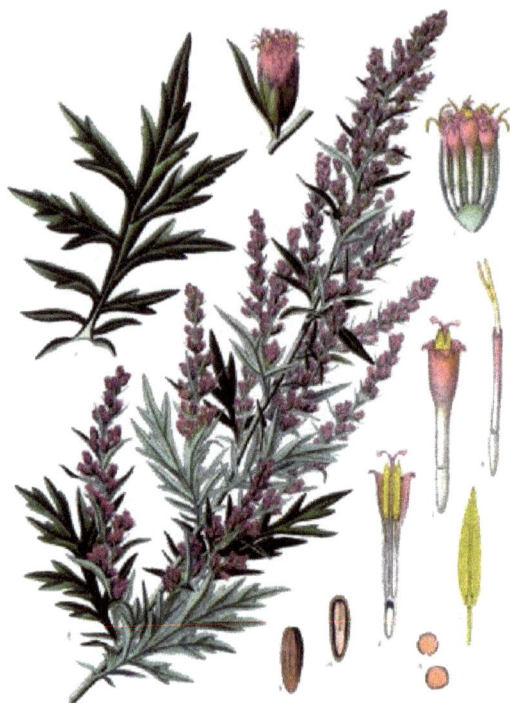

Mugwort, Artemisia vulgaris

(Photo courtesy of commons.wikimedia.org/wiki/
File:Artemisia,vulgaris,-,-016.jpg)

Mugwort is a tall, perennial herb; it can reach up to 1.5 metres in height and has purplish stems. Its leaves are quite distinctive; they vary in size from 2 to 12 cms in length and up to 8 cms in width, with wavy, finger-like lobes along the central vein. The tops of the leaves are smooth and hairless while the undersides possess a soft, silvery-white downiness with numerous small reddish-brown or yellow flowers blooming. It is believed to have originated in East Europe and Western Asia but now grows in temperate climates across the globe. The essential oil is extracted through steam distillation of its dried flower heads.

"This beautiful herb has long been associated with the shadowy world of the seer as well as with the moon".
(Cunningham: p.114)

Like Wormwood, Mugwort is connected to the planet Venus and is sacred to the Goddesses Artemis & Diana and to the Chinese fox spirit Hu Xian. Mugwort is considered to be a visionary herb and grows all over the globe, which probably makes it sacred for many Goddesses.

Mugwort has been used for smudging since ancient times. Its scent is known to be both aromatic and bitter-sweet, and to have the power to clear the atmosphere and promote a sense of calmness. But, it is also from the family of the Artemisia genus, and like the Wormwood plant it is considered toxic because of its Thujone components and the essential oil is rarely used in aromatherapy today. However, it is also used as a fragrance component in soaps, colognes and perfumes.

After years of practising magic, I've realized that the most profound learning and insights into any such work will occur while we are dreaming. Every perfume oil I've created for this book was designed with this in mind, to affect our dreams and alter our minds and our perceptions of nature and the moon cycles in a magical way. I never had a problem remembering my dreams and understanding their meaning and symbolism. Lucid dreaming was one of the skills I learnt early on in life which I refined with age. Working on the Black Magick Perfume/Kurukulla oil evoked a flood of lucid dreaming for several nights in a row.

Both Wormwood and Mugwort are considered witch herbs and in most of the literature I found it is said that both plants will support, strengthen and enhance visualisation, psychic abilities and lucid dreaming. As both plants are dedicated to Venus, the embodiment of all queen witches and black sorceresses, their influence on our psyche will be much greater on the equinoxes or solstices which are the 'in-between' times; the time of the Witches' Sabbat. Kurukulla represents the transitional period, where Lalita's brightness and Kali's darkness are harmonized.

During Kurukulla transitional period, it's a great opportunity to bring in the balancing and harmonizing benefits of Mimosa essential oil. This oil can work wonders when combined with the essential oils we've previously mentioned.

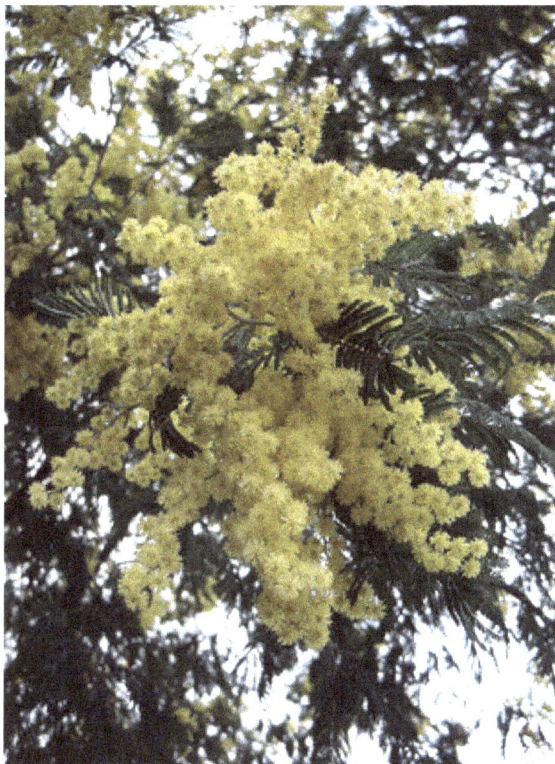

Mimosa, Acacia dealbata

(Photo courtesy of commons.wikimedia.org/wiki/File:Acacia,dealbata-1.jpg)

Acacia dealbata is an attractive tree with a greyish-brown bark and unique longitudinally ridged bark. It has delicate foliage and clusters of fragrant yellow flowers which are harvested for use as cut flowers and referred to in the florist trade as "Mimosa". Widely cultivated in warm temperate regions around the world, Acacia dealbata also grows naturally in southwestern Australia, Norfolk Island, and many of the Mediterranean countries, California, Madagascar, southern Africa, highlands of southern India south-western China and Chile.

Mimosa flowers can add a unique touch in the field of perfumery. Their long-lasting base notes bring harmony to the blend, allowing for a smooth shift from floral and sweet fragrances to earthy and musty scents. This complexity contributes to an alluring scent overall. Mimosa corresponds with the balancing frequency that Kurukulla initiates so we can go deeper and explore the darkest corners of our minds.

Wormwood, Mugwort, and Mimosa essential oil all have a powerful impact on the quality of our slumber. Together they forge a visionary lucid dreaming experience which gives us a peek into the mysteries of the spiritual realm. These three oils encourage deep restorative sleep as well as prophetic dreams.

Adding the Mimosa essence to the blend did soften the herby aroma of Wormwood and Mugwort, but I still sought something that could take it up a notch. I wanted something delicate yet sweet, that would reflect Kurukulla's grace and the powerful work of dark sorcery. So before bedtime, I dabbed on a concoction of Wormwood, Mugwort, and Mimosa and prayed for a dream that would show me the perfect scent. The next day, my dream was clear and vivid.

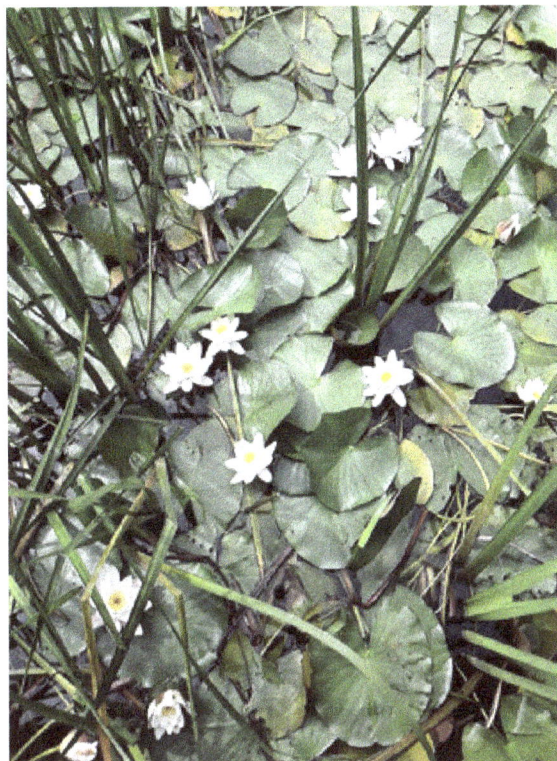

White Lotus, Nymphaea lotus

(Photo by the author)

The white lotus represents mental purity and spiritual perfection. It holds a special place in Hindu philosophy, as it is considered to be the first born of creation and a magical womb for the universe and gods. Its symbolism is far-reaching, and it has been associated with longevity, fertility, wealth, and knowledge. Its beauty is unparalleled, and it is truly a wonder of nature.

For the Egyptians, the White Lotus, which opens shortly after sunset, was a symbol of the Night Sun — the Moon and was considered a symbol of creation and transformation. In the chapter "Black Magick —

Halloween /Samhain/Day of the Dead" I've discussed another aspect of black magic that is less

talked about — the process of growth and regeneration which gives life. Solve et Coagula, is the complete breakdown before we can put it all back together in a better and stronger form. Reflecting on the notion of Solve a Coagula got me thinking about the ancient Egyptian Osiris myth. The Egyptologist Erik Hornung (28 January 1933 – 11 July 2022) was one of the most influential modern writers on ancient Egyptian religion. In his book History of Ancient Egypt: An Introduction (1999), he wrote:

> "Osiris does indeed seem to be absorbed into Ra, and becomes the night sun, which awakens the underworld dwellers from the sleep of death."

White Lotus awakens the essence of the primaeval sorcerers that dwells in the realms of dreams. Its golden sunset colour shines through and illuminates our vision.

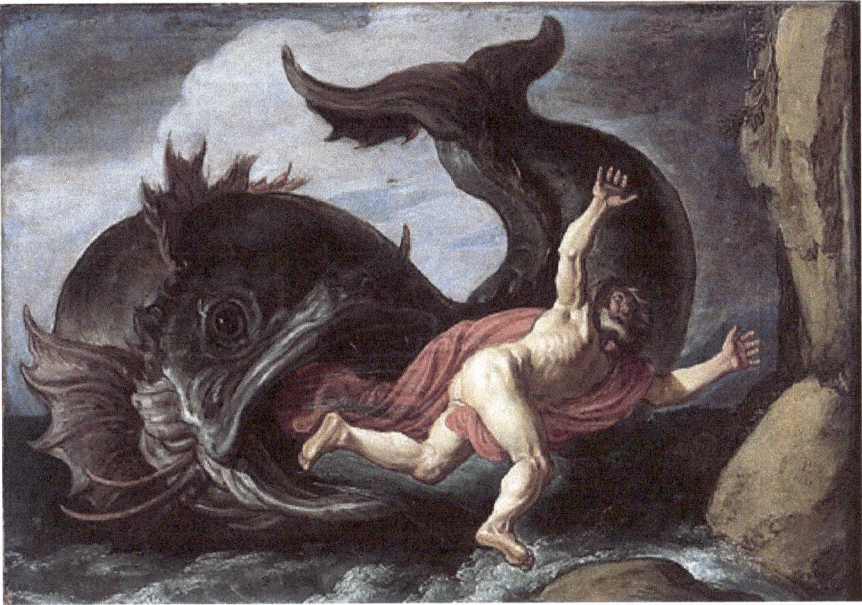

Ambergris

Ambergris is formed from a secretion of the bile duct in the intestines of the sperm whale. wiki image

Ambergris is a waxy substance that is produced in the intestines of sperm whales. It is found primarily in the Atlantic Ocean and on the coasts of South Africa, Brazil, Madagascar, the East Indies, The Maldives, China, Japan, India, Australia, New Zealand and the Molucca Islands. It is used in the manufacture of perfumes. It is interesting to think how little we know about Ambergris despite it being traded since the Middle Ages, yet, it was only recently discovered that it comes from Sperm whales.

The name Ambergris is derived from the old French term ambre gris, which means grey amber. This distinguishes the substance from amber resin, which is fossilized tree sap that can also wash up on beaches and is used in fragrances. Despite their similar names, these two substances actually don't have anything in common.

I find it fascinating that Ambergris can spend years floating on the ocean before it is found. The fact that the longer it is exposed to the sea, the better quality it is thought to be, only adds to the mystery. It is no wonder that it has been considered a unique phenomenon for millennia and has been described as one of the world's strangest natural occurrences. It is usually found in lumps of various shapes and sizes, and weighing from 15 grams to 50 kilograms or more. When initially expelled by or removed from the whale, the fatty precursor of Ambergris is pale white in colour (sometimes streaked with black), soft, and with a strong faecal smell. As it ages, it acquires a sweet, earthy musky scent.

Ambergris oil is a highly valued essential oil, with royal white Ambergris regarded as the pinnacle of quality. Historically, it was used in traditional Chinese medicine and some of the most exclusive perfumes, Ambrein, an odourless alcohol extracted from the substance, was employed to make fragrances last longer. For centuries, the hue of ambergris has been a determining factor when grading its value; pure white being the most precious. Black ambergris on the other hand tends to have less Ambrein thus lesser value.

Laws regulating the collection and sale of Ambergris vary around the world. In some countries, Ambergris and all other whale-derived products are prohibited, but elsewhere it is either legal or a grey area. In most countries including the UK and in the rest of the EU, it is currently perfectly legal to collect a lump of Ambergris, if and when found on beaches and to sell it. However, in the United States, selling and buying Ambergris is illegal because it is obtained from whales, which are endangered species. In India, ambergris is also contraband.

"Hail Leviathan! Hail to the Ancient Serpent! Hail to the Stooping Dragon! Vast, immeasurable and ageless, You coiled through the Void before the worlds were made, You were before time and space were conceived and they are Yours to devour as You will…" (Michael Kelly, *Dragonscales*)

Leviathan – לִוְיָתָן , in Hebrew means Whale. Leviathan represents the primal (sea) dragon. From very early in human history, our mythologies were full of primal dragons and serpents. The Sumerian Tiamat, Nun and Apep of ancient Egypt, the Dragon Fafnir from the Sagas of the Northern Tradition, the four ancient Chinese mythological dragons: the Celestial Dragon (Tianlong), who guards the heavenly dwellings of the gods; the Dragon of Hidden Treasure (Fuzanglong); the Earth Dragon (Dilong), who controls the waterways; and the Spiritual Dragon (Shenlong), who controls the rain and winds. There are many more dragons around the world that I haven't mentioned here, it would require writing a whole book to include them all.

When I think about Leviathan, I can't help but recall the story of Jonah who was swallowed by a large fish. He spent three days and three nights in the fish's belly. While inside the fish, Jonah prayed to God in his affliction and promised to give thanks. God then commanded the fish to vomit Jonah out.

The belly of Leviathan symbolises the abyss we are standing before. Once swallowed or devoured by Leviathan, we are heading full power into that abyss, knowing that the only way out is through Leviathan's digestive system. This is our signal to wake up and take responsibility for our actions. The experiences of being in a trying circumstance (within Leviathan) help us gain a deeper understanding of the roads traversed and the ones still to come. Once we acknowledge the facts, and register their impact on our innermost self, it is as if we become a part of Leviathan's contents, like the precious Ambergris we are waiting to be purged and transformed into something far greater. We emerge renewed, with a new outlook on life.

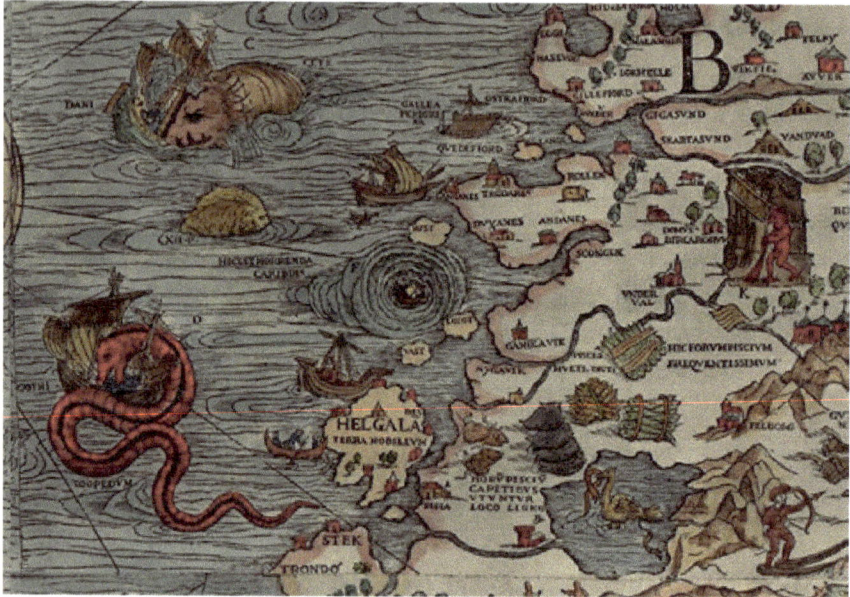

Carta Marina (Photo courtesy of commons.wikimedia.org/wiki/File:Maelstrom,Carta,Marina.png)

HC SVNT DRACONES,

"Here will be Dragons"

Dragons are the substance of our dreams that manifest our magical reality.

The Triune brain theory, developed by Paul MacLean, is a landmark model that sections the brain into three distinct parts. The most ancient part of our brain, the reptilian brain, holds sway over essential physiological mechanisms such as the respiratory rate, heartbeat and temperature regulation. This foundation is formed of structures commonly found in reptiles: the brainstem and cerebellum. Our reptilian brain can be quite reliable but also inflexible and overly structured.

Dragons are commonly depicted as having dominion over the primordial Chaos before the Universe came to be, existing outside of time and space. This is very much the playground of Lalita and her daughters, the Kalas, each one of them represents a moment that exists outside of our normal perception of time and space.

In her wonderful book *Earthsea*, Ursula K. Le Guin wrote: "The dragons do not dream. They are dreams. They do not work magic: it is their substance, their being. They do not do: they are."

Kurukulla awakens within us the memory of the ancient She-Dragon, the "built-in" reptilian brain we are all sharing. Her essence is of the precious Ambergris which comes from the depth of her reality. And just like her, its beauty and its secrets will develop, be appreciated and understood with the passing of time.

8. Waning Moon

"We use breath retention in our asana practice to intensify the effects of a posture" (Desikachar p.38)

In yoga, the process of inhalation and exhalation can be compared to the phases of the moon. At the new moon, we start a fresh cycle with a lengthy inhalation ? 'brahmana', which translates as 'expansion'. As the waxing moon takes form, we pause briefly and hold our breath in observance. We are witnessing the evolution of our new projects, developing shape and direction.

At the full moon, we practice 'aghana' ? a long exhalation which all about reducing or fasting. This lasts until the waning moon when we pause and assess if anything remains to be breathed out. With this, all notions and intentions taken in upon the new moon are released. The relevance of 'aghana' is to make room on our following inhalation for fresh plans and ideas to be ingested upon the upcoming new moon.

"Only when we have emptied ourselves can we take in a new breath" (Desikachar p.60)

"Holding the breath actually gives us a moment in which nothing happens ..." "It is even said that the best moment for introducing a mantra is not the inhalation or the exhalation, but while you are holding the breath ..." "It is said that a moment of breath retention is a moment of meditation, a moment of dhyana". (Desikachar p.67)

On the night of the waning moon, we meet with Ugra – 'The hungry one', 'The Fearful', 'She who brings us to the shore' – the shores of realization, of knowledge. The waning is a cosmic time in the cycle of the moon, when we stop and hold our breath and recite the mantra for Ugra:

Om svim hum hrim hum phat svaha

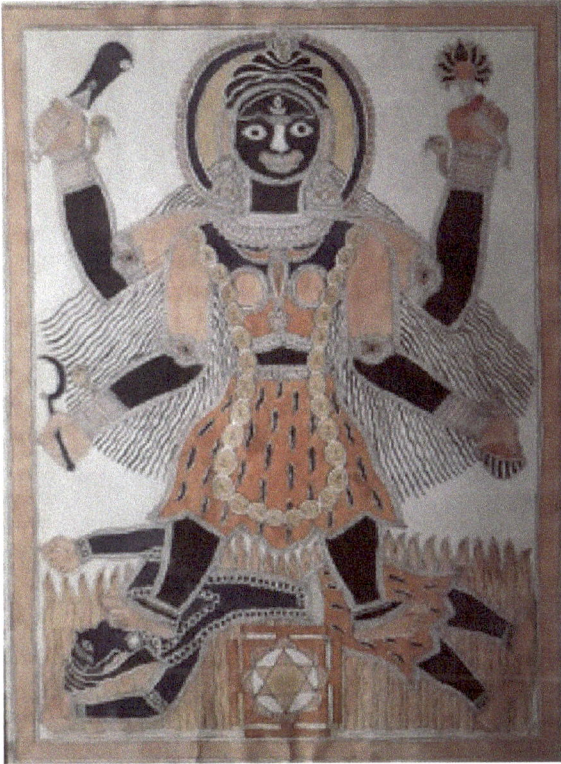

(Ugra, print on fabric, author's collection)

Ugra

"Nothing exists but by devouring something else". "In the waste of the boundless all-devouring Time, the all-devouring hunger appears". "The Power of Hunger".

(Alain Danielou, *The Myths and Gods of India*)

Seven days after the full moon, the flow of the moonblood is nearly gone or finished. Any blood after that point will remind us of our painful attachment to the old. The last drops of the moonblood remind us of our attachments to the past, our resentment of change and our breaking of the ties of old.

The waning moon is a fleeting moment in time, that offers us a cosmic window of opportunity to be courageous, embrace change, and move forward by shedding our old selves.

Like the eternal serpent, the Ouroboros, the endometrial tissue is shedding its 'skin' month after month. During the night of the waning moon, Ugra reminds us that Kali's cycle is halfway through and that the light will soon fade into complete darkness. The final quarter of the waning moon is an opportune moment to offer something to the 'hungry one' and request that she grant us what we truly desire. Kali, the goddess of time, generously grants us another moment to seize and make the most of. Be wise of what you ask of the goddess, as on the following night she will be back, this time as Ugraprabha, who represents Kali in all her aspects; creator and benefactor, destroyer and the personification of time, space, knowledge and eternal light, known in Hebrew as the 'Ein Sof Or'.

The primary distinguishing factors between Kali and Ugra are their implements and colours. Ugra is typically black and possesses a sacrificial sword, a severed head or skull cup, a blue lotus, and a flaying knife, while Kali never carries a lotus or a flaying knife and is depicted in blue.

According to the Adbhuta version of the Indian epic the Ramayana, after Sita, in the form of Kali, slew the demon Ravana Brahma, she assumed the calmer form of Tara. Rudra (Shiva) lay on the ground and requested the boon of Brahmavidya (knowledge) from her, to which she responded by placing her left foot on his chest and enlightening him. As thanks, Shiva offered her a blue lotus and a skull cup. As previously mentioned, the Kapala serves as a sacred vessel for spiritual metamorphosis, where all hindrances and toxins are poured and transmuted into divine nectar. By gifting Kali the skull cup, Shiva is sharing the secrets of "churning the ocean". Churning of the Ocean is a mythical story of Hinduism and Hindu mythology. Vasuki, the serpent is pulled back and forth and starts churning the ocean. Poison escapes from Vasuki's mouth and this terrifies both the Gods and demons, as it was lethal enough to destroy everything. The Gods approach Lord Shiva for protection and he consumes this poison to save the Universe.

The Kapala, also known as the skull cup, signifies the transformation of poison into the divine nectar of immortality. Meanwhile, the lotus flower is often regarded as sacred due to its ability to remain pure even when growing in muddy waters. The Blue Lotus is associated with wisdom and intelligence and is typically depicted with its petals slightly open. Shiva's gift of the Blue Lotus denotes the continual growth and evolution of the wisdom possessed by its recipient. On the night of the waning moon, Ugra offers us the boons of transformation, growth and Knowledge and a chance to feed our spiritual hunger.

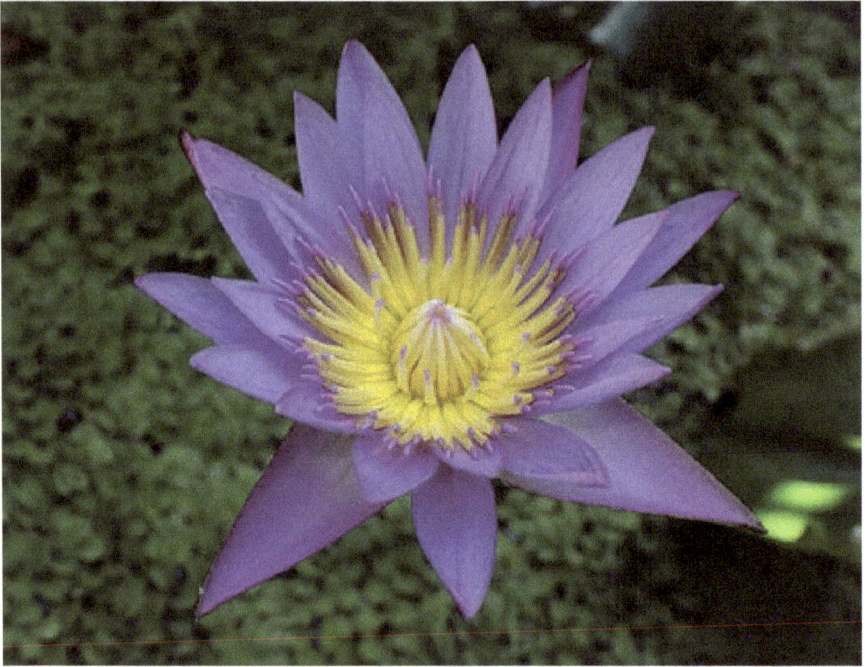

Blue lotus, Nymphaea nouchali

(Photo courtesy of commons.wikimedia.org/wiki/
File:Nymphaea,nouchali,kz04.jpg

Nymphaea nouchali is a water lily of the genus Nymphaea. It is native to southern and eastern parts of Asia and is the national flower of Bangladesh and Sri Lanka. It is often known by its common names Blue Lotus, Star Lotus, Dwarf Aquarium Lily, Blue Water Lily, Blue Star Water Lily or Manel Flower. In Sanskrit, it is Utpala. This species is usually considered to include the blue Egyptian lotus N. nouchali var. Caerulea. The oil is extracted from the flower by solvent extraction.

The unfolding petals of the Blue Lotus flower suggest the soul's expansion. The growth of its pure beauty from the mud of its origin holds a spiritual promise. When Shiva requested the gift of knowledge from Kali, he embraced the thirst for knowledge that permeates the vast conscious universe. This is the same hunger that drives us to create art, music and life. The hunger that ignites in our hearts the passion to study and learn science, medicine, alchemy, philosophy and magic. Ugra represents the darker form of Kali, hence her name Ugra 'The Terrible', The Formidable or Enchantress of Terrifying Form. She appears naked, black-skinned, with large fangs and blood dripping from her mouth. (Gregory Peters: Yogini Magic). The symbolism of the blue lotus and the skull cup in her possession implies that she possesses the ability to transform and manipulate any toxic substance, utilising it to satisfy her insatiable thirst for spiritual enlightenment.

The Blue water lily or lotus, is an aquatic plant that mostly grows in Egypt and certain parts of Asia. The lotus plant contains many flavonoids, terpenoids, and alkaloids compounds that may act as antioxidants, fight inflammation and act as an antibacterial agent. The blue Egyptian lotus N. nouchali var. Caerulea contains two alkaloids apomorphine and nuciferine that stimulate dopamine receptors which affect movements, rewards, and emotions in the brain.

In both Egyptian and Hindu cultures, the Blue Lotus is well known for promoting spiritual growth, healing, balancing and rejuvenation. Antioxidants are essential in fighting against oxidation and the production of free radicals, which can harm organic compounds - including living organisms. By scavenging for these destructive particles, they are able to decrease and stop the damage they cause. Not only do antioxidants protect from radical harm, but also promote healthy skin by manipulating intracellular signals responsible for skin cell damage and guarding against photodamage. Plus, they help restore skin damage as inflammation can block the renewal progress. Antioxidants have the ability to reduce inflammation, allowing the skin to repair itself while also getting rid of any visible damage. Certain antioxidants even encourage collagen production, required for achieving younger-looking and revitalized skin.

Shiva's offering of the Blue Lotus highlights its profound history as a healing plant in Indian Ayurvedic medicine. The complex compounds present in the Blue lotus are known to provide soothing and calming effects, helping us to unwind and relax muscle spasms while providing a sense of euphoria.

The captivating scent of Blue Lotus Absolute essential oil is truly one-of-a-kind. Blending together warm, spicy, sweet, and floral notes all at once, the fragrance has a complex intensity that is perfectly balanced with subtle refinement. The Egyptians and Hindus of ancient times believed that such exquisite smells were signs of the divine's presence – symbols of transformation and rebirth. This theory has been extended to suggest that fragrances can shape our mental and emotional states as well. Upon first inhalation, Blue Lotus evokes a sense of longing for both the past and future; love is not far away. As the aroma fills your senses, they become filled with pure pleasure and appreciation for the physical world's beauty. And with every breath, an overwhelming sense of euphoria begins to take hold – comforting us like a hug from the Goddess herself.

Ugraprabha

On the 8th night of the dark half, we encounter Ugraprabha - "the magnificent one" and the "wrathful resplendent goddess" (Yogini Magic). Unlike her sister Ugra, her skin is Blue. All impediments have been eliminated and she is now complete. Appearing with the head of a fox, this beguiling Yogini can entrance you with her grin. She presides over seminal fluids and pleasures of the flesh and carries the euphoric scent of Blue Lotus. She bestows upon us sexual magic as a boon.

Ugra & Ugraprabha Ritual bath

¼ cup oats

¼ cup Blue Lily dried flowers

1 tablespoon of sea/Himalaya/Epsom salt

1 teaspoon almond oil

2-3 drops Blue Lily essential oil.

Blend all the components in a little bowl and inhale the captivating aroma of Blue Lily. Let it pervade your heart with affection and extend your awareness. Finally, add the mixture to your bath water.

Cult of the Hidden God

(Excerpt from Mogg Morgan, *Aleister Crowley & Thelemic Magick*)

There is also said to be a secret method by which the phases of the moon are somehow 'controlled' or predicted by Seth's northern constellation Ursa major, The Plough etc. But the primary lunar reference comes from the fact that in myth, Seth dismembers the first king Osiris into 14 or 15 pieces.

Fourteen or fifteen days could be a half lunation — so it seems likely that what we are seeing here is a very ancient system of correspondences between the parts of the moon and the human body. I've argued elsewhere that the contention found in several authors, including Kenneth Grant's, of some kind of parallel between the Tantrik doctrine of the Kalas or lunar phases and its earlier Egyptian model is essentially correct. In fact it seems highly likely that many of the secret body magick techniques of the ancient Egyptians were transferred or certainly only survived in India, after the systematic destruction of the Egyptian religion and sacred technologies by Christianity.

In the courtly erotic texts such as the Kama Sutra there are laid out certain doctrines. Before I go on to describe them — a couple of points are worthy of note.

Occult tradition from Egyptian times states that the moon has four phases. The fourth phase is rarely talked about in books but is reserved as secret knowledge to be transmitted orally. Incidentally you might consider what happens to the Tarot if you add five 'hidden' cards of the major arcana? This has led to the common misunderstanding that the moon is threefold. It has been said that the so-called triple goddess of 'virgin/maiden, mother, crone' does not represent a very positive set of female archetypes. Some would say the three — virgin, mother, crone are the three times in a woman's life when she has least fun — sexually that is. Others that they represent the least empowered aspects of a woman's life.

The elision of the fourth phase is especially interesting. Four is in many cultures an inauspicious number. It is often used to designate the fourth and most heterodox part of a system. Hence the fourth Veda — the Atharva is the most magical and diverse. The 'fourth' Book of Occult Philosophy — the 'fourth' Book of the Law. So the fourth phase of anything, is from a particular perspective likely to be the most interesting. In Egyptian cosmology there was a fourth or 'secret' region, called Setaue and conceived as being behind the seven stars of the Big Dipper and therefore ruled by Seth, (Webb p.34). Sokar, an early form of Osiris was called the 'lord of the mouth of the passages to this secret place, ie some connection here between Setaue and fear of initiation.

The fourth lunar stage is the dark waning moon, the moon's final quarter — and perhaps as an archetype this is the 'scarlet woman' — she may physically be either of the other three, i.e. a virgin, a mother or even an older woman — but in a sense she stands outside of these as a woman in her own right.

You might struggle hard to find a goddess to fill this role — most traditional love goddesses of the past don't quite do it — with the possible exception of Seth's sometime consort Nephthys. The response of modern magi is to make one up — hence Babalon.

The term 'Kala' as found in the works of Kenneth Grant, is a Sanskrit term meaning part or digit. There is a maxim in Hinduism that 'Man is a microcosm of the universe — as above so below'. Sound familiar? This is pretty much identical to the Hermetic doctrine of the so-called Emerald Tablet. So if the physical moon can be described as having 28 or 30 different parts or phases throughout the month, half waxing, half waning. Then these parts are also reflected in the subtle anatomy of every human being. This Tantrik system is not to be confused with the system of talismanic magick based on the lunar mansions popular in grimoires from the time of Pope Honorius until about the time of Francis Barrett when it fell into disuse.

These 28 or 30 parts are most noticeable in the doctrine of erogenous zones (chandrakala) — zones of sensitivity that migrate around the body through the course of a month.

9. The Dark Moon

The dark moon invites stillness and encourages us to reflect on our actions over the last month, releasing any that did not serve us. We can use this time to set our intentions for the upcoming new moon cycle. To comprehend the depths of darkness that the moon can bring, one must keep watch on the last day of the month when it fades from sight and hides itself away, leaving us in a state of absolute blackness.

Mita, associated with the dark moon, marks the end of the phase which had begun with Kula, the third Kala in the Kali sequence. She embodies the very fabric of the universe and our comprehension, largely rooted in the concepts of time and space, cause and effect. Kula reminds us of the idea that "All is one" and its journey through the 'Ein Sof Or' אין סוף אור – The Infinite Light. Kula marks the commencement of the lunar cycle's decline and illustrates how to connect to the source of infinite light found within each Kalas in the Kali sequence.

On the darkest night of the month, Mita 'The Measurer', determines the time, location, causation, action and outcome. Armed with her findings, she embarks on a new cycle; and so do we.

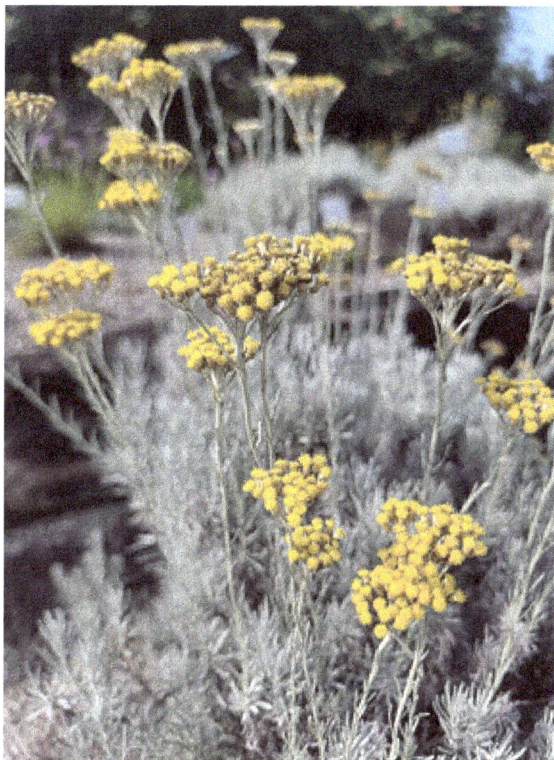

Helichrysum, *Helichrysum angustifolium*

(Photo courtesy of commons.wikimedia.org:
Helichrysum italicum in Kyoto.jpg)

The name Helichrysum has its roots in the Greek words helisso and chrysos, respectively meaning Sun and gold. It is also commonly referred to as Immortelle or Everlasting, aptly reflecting its remarkable qualities and benefits. This plant's healing properties are drawn from the immutability of the Sun's gold. Mita The Measurer brings forth the seed of the infinite light that is at the heart of the darkest night of the month with the knowledge that one measure has come to an end while the next one is about to start anew.

The everlasting nature of Helichrysum can teach us about the immortality of the soul and the mysteries of self-regeneration.

Helichrysum is a herbaceous plant of light green or silvery hue, reaching up to 60cm in height. With its bright yellow blooms that don't lose their colour when dried, it has earned the name 'everlasting'. Native to the Mediterranean and North Africa areas, its scent can be either sweet and floral or even resemble honey and fruit. Throughout history, Helichrysum oil has been a key part of any skincare routine, whether it is in cosmetic blends designed for wrinkles or mature skin, or to soothe inflamed skin conditions, scars or burns. Not only that, this amazing plant can help our mental health too - helping us move past old pain and open up a new journey of healing by letting go of the past.

Dark Moon (Bath) ritual

For the ritual, you will need a mirror, a candle and helichrysum essential oil and calendula flowers (In case you cannot find helichrysum oil you can substitute it with calendula oil or flowers).

Mix together a tablespoon of sea or Epsom salt and 3-5 drops of helichrysum oil in a little bowl. As an alternative, you can add one teaspoon of calendula oil to the bath instead of this blend. You may also want to toss in a few dried calendula flowers.

Before you get into the bath, dim the lights in the room you are in and light the candle. Sit or stand in front of a mirror or hold it in your hand. Take a couple of deep breaths and stare into your eyes which are reflected back at you from the mirror.

Say the following words 3 times:
The moon's darkness swallows the sky, Mita, the measurer, is in charge tonight. What does she measure, you might ask? She measures the depth of my darkness for tomorrow, the new moon will rise and the measure of darkness will be the same as that of light.

When your bath is full, add the contents of the bowl into it and move your hand in a figure-eight pattern as you concentrate on your intentions.

Once you're submerged in the bath, let your body relax in the water. Close your eyes and inhale deeply, absorbing the aroma of the oil and say:

I honour the dark moon and release my body unto it.

Inhale deeply and on the exhalation, release your intentions for the upcoming month.

Mahakali

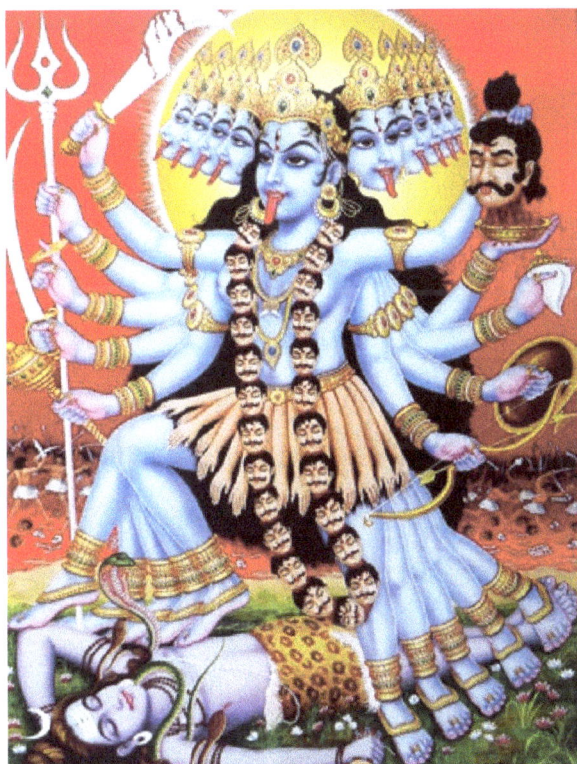

(Mahakali Dasmukhi by Mukesh 'a god photograph',
printed by Brijbasi, author's collection)

She is said to embody the 10 Mahavidyas (great wisdom), portrayed with 10 heads, 10 arms and 10 legs.

The dark moon is a reminder of the importance of balance between luminosity and obscurity. It signifies Kali, who brings to light the brilliance of Lalita and Mita, which measure the immense darkness that Mahakali radiates. Mahakali, which translates to 'Great Kali' in English, is the Goddess of time, life and death. The 16th Kala appears in both Shakti and Kali's sequence; Lalita denotes all creation and manifestation in the light sequence, whereas Mahakali stands for the perpetual cycle of liberation, rebirth and transformation in the dark sequence. Mahakali is accompanied by a black jackal, hyena and raven which are symbols of the unknown, messengers from the spirit realm and omens of dreams, premonitions and insight. Life begins in darkness. The initial steps towards a new chapter are evident as Mita has taken the initiative and sowed them deep in our psyches beneath Mahakali's veil. Tonight, our dreams will give us a sign or a clue of how to nurture and cultivate the Kala mandala, allowing us to expand, evolve and become everlastingly linked with the Lunar Flowers' essence.

Part II
Eight Witches Sabbaths
and
The Eight Colours of Magick

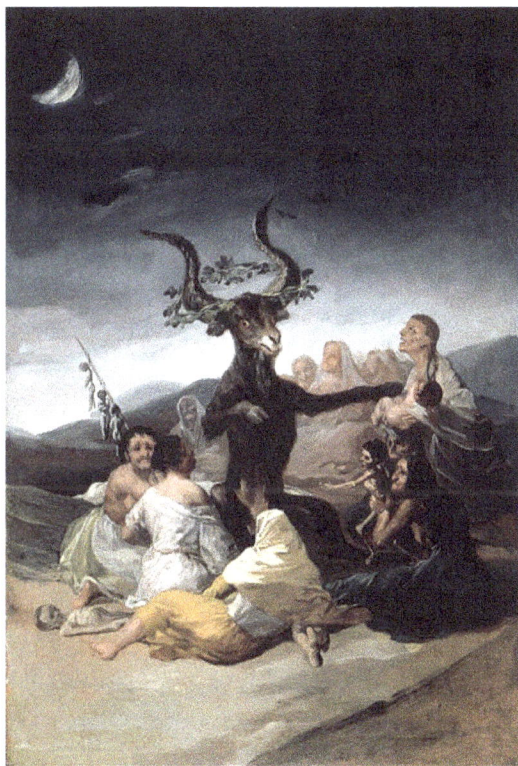

Francisco de Goya 'Witches Sabbath'
(Photo courtesy of wiki commons wikimedia.org)

Rap to Pan

Thrill with lovely lust of the light,

O man! My man!

Come charging out of the night

Of Pan! Io Pan!

Io Pan! Io Pan! Come over the sea

From Shambala and paradise !

Roaming like Bacchus, with his guards

Companion females and males all hard

On a milk-white ass, come over the sea

To me, to me!

Come with a priestess in bridal dress

(Shepherdess and pythoness)

Come with Artemis, who in wildwood trod,

And wash your white thigh, beautiful god,

In the moon of the woods, on the lotus press,

The golden tongue my jewel to bless!

Dip the purple of passionate prayer

In the crimson shrine, lusty & bare,

Your soul that startles with eyes of blue

As we watch your ecstasy seeping through

The tangled thicket, the ancient grove

Of the living tree that is spirit and soul

And body and brain — come over the sea,

(Io Pan! Io Pan!)

Devil or god, to me, to me,

My man! my man!

Come with trumpets sounding shrill

Over the hill!

Come with drums low thundering

From the spring!

Come with a flute and come with a pipe!

Am I not ripe?

I, who wait and tremble and wrestle

With breathe that has no way to settle

My body, weary of empty embrace,

Strong as a lion and smooth as a snake —

Come, O come!

I am numb

With the lonely lust of devildom.

Thrust the sword through iron fetters,

All-devourer, all-begetter;

Give me the sign of the Open Eye,

And the token aroused of horny thigh,

And the word of madness and mystery,

O Pan! Io Pan!

Io Pan! Io Pan Pan! Pan Pan! Pan,

I am one love

Do as you will, as a great god can,

O Pan! Io Pan!

Io Pan! Io Pan Pan! I am awake

In the grip of the snake.

The eagle slashes with beak and claw;

The gods withdraw:

The great beasts come. Io Pan! I am borne

To come on the horn

Of the Unicorn.

I am Pan! Io Pan! Io Pan Pan! Pan!

I am your mate, I am your one,

Goat of your flock, I am gold, I am god,

Flesh to your bone, flower to your rod.

With hoofs of steel, I race on the rocks

Through solstice sunrise to equinox.

And I rave, and I howl and I rip and I rend

Everlasting, world without end,

Maenad, Mystoi, Woman, Man,

In the might of Pan.

Io Pan! Io Pan Pan! Pan! Io Pan!

(Minanath 2018 - found after AC)

10. Eight Sabbaths and Eight Colours

According to Peter Carroll, *Liber Kaos* – "Our perceptual and conceptual apparatus creates a fourfold division of matter into the space, time, mass, and energy tautology. Similarly, our instinctual drives create an eightfold division of magic. The eight forms of magic are conveniently denoted by colours having emotional significance"

In the magical system of Chaos Craft (check out *Chaos Craft* by Julian Vayne & Steve Dee), the eight magics and their colours are assigned to each of the witch's sabbath. As a witch, I follow this current, and I could not notice the resonance of the colours and essences with each turn of the year's wheel was unavoidable.

Going deeper, you can orient your work around the eight sabbaths of the year and their colours, appreciating the Kala that resides over each sabbath and enhances the energies of that particular day and night. You will find that each year, the Kalas will vary slightly as the cycle of the moon is in constant motion.

The Eight Colours of Magics

Octarine – winter solstice

Green – Imbolc

Orange – Spring equinox

Purple – Beltane

Yellow – Summer solstice

Red – Lammas/Lughnasadh

Blue – Autumn equinox - Mabon

Black – Halloween/Samhain/Day of the Dead

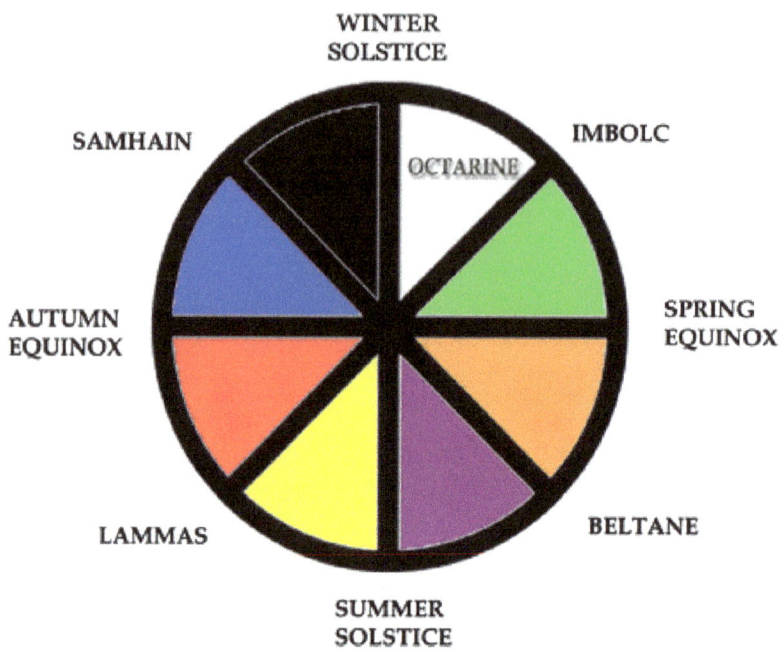

WINTER
SOLSTICE

SAMHAIN

IMBOLC

OCTARINE

AUTUMN
EQUINOX

SPRING
EQUINOX

LAMMAS

BELTANE

SUMMER
SOLSTICE

11. Octarine Magick
Winter Solstice

When wandering in ignorance
Seeking the Enlightenment of Universal Consciousness
May the Light inspire and strengthen me
May the Divine Mother comfort and sustain me
May I be spared a long and painful transition
May I be one with the Central Realm
Of Universal Consciousness
From *The NU Tantras of the Uttarakaulas* by John Power

Twice a year, on the winter and summer solstice, a very unique portal reveals itself. Through this opening, we are given the opportunity to explore both the chill, yet still spirit of tranquillity and the effervescent radiance of brightness.

In *The Book of Thoth* (1944) Crowley wrote:

"...deep indigo, the colour of Saturn, the Lord of Time."

The deep, indigo night sky of the winter solstice is reminiscent of Saturn, Lord of Time. There is something special about its seemingly timeless journey; almost as though time actually has stopped. The winter solstice marks the occasion when the Earth's axis reaches its highest angle away from the Sun.

In the Northern Hemisphere, this is where we observe the least amount of sunlight, leading to a day that's shorter than any other of the year and a night that's longer. This day mirrors the symbolic death and rebirth of the Sun— with daylight hours beginning to grow again afterwards.

You fair, united, through a gate called seat of her lord,
Guarded by a Serpent, He whose eye roves about.
Mind says: "Open the door for Ra,
Throw open the door for the One of the Horizon,
He lightens the complete darkness,
And makes the Hidden Chamber bright."
You and the God sail through,
On the winding waterway,
The great door closes after you,
Which makes the dead souls wail.
(from *Egyptian Magick* by Mogg Morgan)

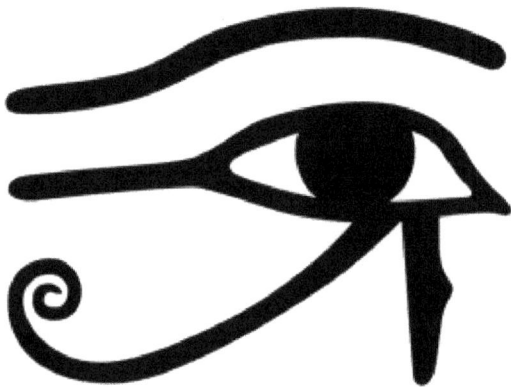

Octarine is the so-called Colour of Magic or King Colour, only perceivable by magicians and cats. According to Discworld texts (see Terry Pratchett's The Colour of Magic), it is a combination of fluorescent greenish yellow and purple, mixing all primary colours, and serves as a representation of imagination.

Octarine Gnosis

The Ancient Romans linked Chronos with Saturn, a deity in their own pantheon. Chronos was one of three gods that represented the idea of time within Greek mythology — alongside Aion and Kairos.

Chronos represented the essence of linear time as known and experienced: Birth - Life - Death.

Aion represented eternal time and was associated with the afterlife and the cyclical nature of certain events (e.g. the seasons).

Kairos was considered the embodiment of opportunist time. Specifically, moments when action must be taken to achieve a task. (Michael Roy: 2020)

At the winter solstice, we meet the three Timelords, Chronos and Aion have brought us to this special evening, this gateway.

We must unlock what lies ahead by connecting to Kairos and capturing the various possibilities that lie beyond the gate of transformation, kindling our inner spark of radiance.

Be forewarned, interacting with the Timelords may take you on an adventurous journey of unbelievable highs and lows. If you're fortunate enough, you could even witness a supernova.

The Hierophant

The Hierophant

Crowley's Thoth Tarot offers a much richer layer of meanings and symbolism than usual. His underlying messages convey his ideas and beliefs, making the deck an intriguing source for contemplation. Prior to analyzing the symbolism of this card, we'll only consider it from a Crowlian perspective — namely, my own. To get a better grasp of the Hierophant, let's first look at what it signifies. The Hierophant is a person, often a priest, who deciphers spiritual secrets or arcane doctrines. As a Hierophant, one brings the congregation into an awe-inspiring presence and interprets spiritual secrets and obscure principles. Particularly at the Eleusinian Mysteries in Attica, this role was held within the Philaidae or Eumolpidae families. Hierophant and High Priestess were of equal status, with the responsibility of embodying Demeter and Persephone respectively in ritual.

From the above, we can understand that the hierophant is a top religious figure like the Pope, or the chief Rabbi, whose job was to be a conductor, a channel, funnel or mediator between the gods and the people. In this particular card, focusing only on the hidden symbolism, the hierophant is the representation of the goddess Nuit.

Nuit is the embodiment of infinite space and also the mother of all stars — for it's known that "Every man and every woman is a star"(*Liber AL*, chapter 1, verse 3). With this in mind, she is where each star returns. Additionally, she is also the divine law which must be given to those who follow the hierophant.

"Let the woman be girt with a sword before me" (*Liber AL*, chapter 3, verse 11) At the front of the card, before the hierophant, we can see the woman girt with a sword. *The Book of Thoth* speaks of the 'Scarlet Woman' as an emblem of the new era; she stands for a transformation away from her traditional image as a housewife or accessory to her male partner, instead embracing her identity while searching for autonomy and equality. We can see how all of this manifests in the MeToo movement of our days.

> "The woman is the priestess; in her reposes the mystery. She is the mother, brooding yet tender; the lover, at once passionate and aloof; the wife, revered and cherished. She is the witch woman." (*Freedom is a Two-edged Sword*, Jack Parsons)

The deeper we look into the hidden symbolism and meaning of this mysterious woman, the clearer it becomes that she can be Nuit herself, guarding the divine law. The law is simple and clear and the hierophant's job is to pass it to their congregation:

"Do what thou wilt shall be the whole of the Law"

"Love is the law, love under will"

Or in our words:

"Love and do what you will."

"The symbolism of the Wand is peculiar" – Solve et Coagula (Aleister Crowley, *The Book of Thoth*). Crowley describes the three interlaced rings of the wand, as a "representative of the three Aeons of Isis, Osiris and Horus". However, on a closer look, we see that the hierophant holding the wand with its three rings aspiring upward, in his right hand (solve).

As a Setian/Typhonian, I couldn't help the thought that the three interlaced rings would be much more comfortable in the right hand of destruction (solve) as a representative of Set, Osiris & Ra.

Set and Osiris are both Ra's grandsons and make a sacred triad. Both brothers have to sacrifice themselves for the continuation of Ra — of life — Osiris by being killed by his brother Set, and Set killing his brother and becoming the 'outcast' God.

The demonstration of the cycle of life through destruction and creation is continued with the symbolism of the hierophant's left hand. His left hand (coagula) is pointing downward in the Shamak mudra hand position. I must admit that this never occurred to me before, but once I became aware of it, I could not un-see it. The Shamak mudra, also called the kidney mudra, is the perfect hand position to deliver the message of Solve et Coagula (destruction and creation). At the start, I had difficulty understanding how the Shamak mudra was linked with Solve et Coagula and its role in occult symbology in particular for the hierophant and his wand.

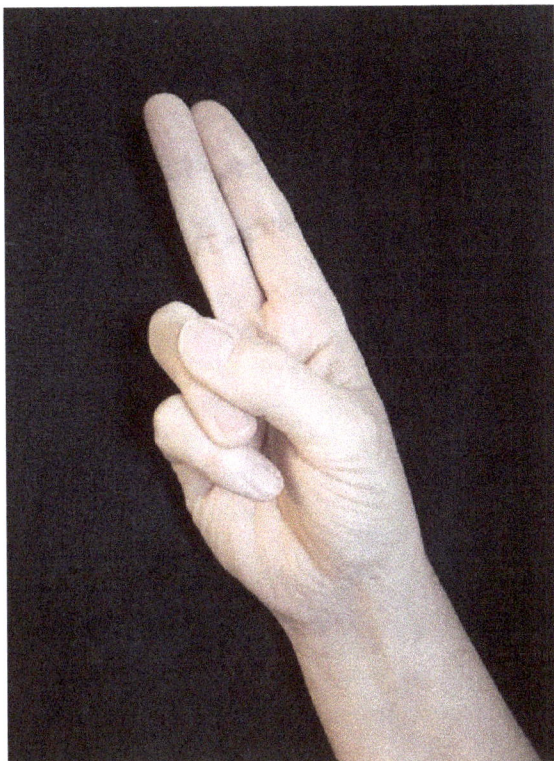

Shamak mudra

Coagulation means the action or process of a liquid, especially blood, changing to a solid or semi-solid state. (OED)

The main function of the kidneys is to cleanse the blood of toxins and transform the waste into urine. The hierophant's right hand in the Shamak mudra, suggests that before we can coagulate, we must be cleansed and purified of all toxins. Only then can we coagulate into our new and transformed selves.

"The Throne of the Hierophant is surrounded by elephants, which are of the nature of Taurus; and he is actually seated upon a bull." (Aleister Crowley, The Book of Thoth). At first sight, the card seems to resonate with the symbolism of the zodiac sign Taurus, which is an earth sign.

The element of earth is represented in this card as the Bull/Kerub and symbolises the earth element at its most balanced and strong. If we look at the symbolism of the bull from the Setian perspective, it takes us back to the prehistoric 'cattle cult', which is probably one of the world's oldest.

Egyptian male deities often have a bull representation. Set is most notably known for the 'Bull of Ombos'. It is likely that this bull cult evolved out of the Cattle cult, which was centred around the Heavenly Cow/Hathor, who symbolizes the feminine aspect of this tradition.

The bull is associated with male fertility and strength, seen in energy, stamina and endurance. Worshipped in antiquity, it is also linked to the zodiac sign Taurus, which is associated with spring in the agricultural calendar as a symbol of renewal, prosperity and abundance. However, this powerful creature can be equally connected to hard-headedness,

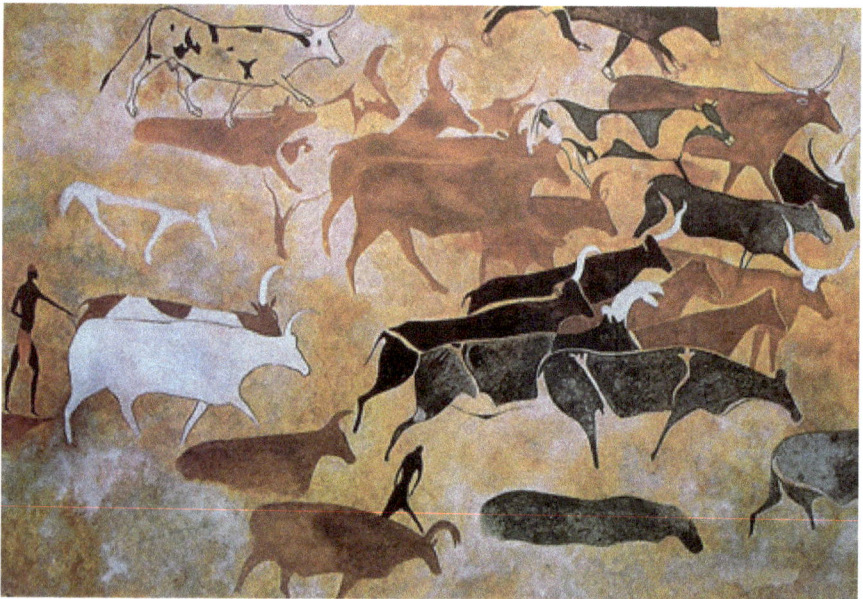

Cave paintings from the Tassili n'Ajjer mountains
(photo courtesy of wiki commons wikimedia.org)

ferocity and brutality — all the qualities of a deity — where it would accept a sacrificial offering as an act of reverence. It is easy to believe that religious reverence for the bull's cult has been forgotten in modern times, yet our practices today have still taken on a new form - the dairy and meat industry.

Just to remind you, a hierophant is a person who brings religious congregants into the presence of that which is deemed holy. As such, a hierophant interprets sacred mysteries and arcane principles. In this card, the hierophant symbolises the link to the secret of the rhythm of time and the ancient practice of the worship of the bull.

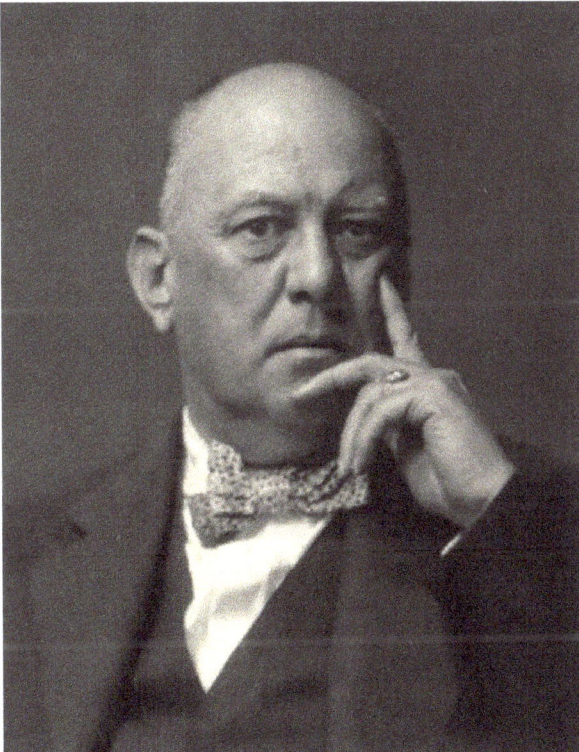

A Timelord (Photo courtesy of wiki commons wikimedia.org)

The secrets of the Timelords are encoded in the divine law which is guarded by Nuit/Nwt and delivered by the hierophant.

The Octarine power lies within us, kindling the spark of the magician self in our inner being. When this flame is lit, we become familiar with various god forms, such as Baphomet, which can be summoned to inspire our magical creativity.

Invocation

In the first aeon, I was the Great Spirit
In the second aeon, Men knew me as the Horned God, Pangenitor Panphage
In the third aeon, I was the Dark One, the Devil
In the fourth aeon, Men know me not, for I am the Hidden One
In this new aeon, I appear before you as Baphomet The God before all gods who shall endure to the end of the Earth.
Peter J. Carroll, *Liber Null & Psychonaut*

The essence of Baphomet restores the balance of our universe.

I see Baphomet as a symbol of equilibrium between all living things. This consciousness allows us to recognize and embrace the connection between humans, mammals, reptiles, fish, angels and demons, heaven and earth. It also encourages us to accept the innate cycle of life and death, plus the concept of eternity. Light and dark, left and right; these are all balanced by Baphomet's equanimity. I found it easier to identify with Baphomet consciousness when I think of it as a model for a unique and original thought, a primal idea of balance. This concept once initiated, will ignite the flames of a passionate heart and open a clear passage for communication with our higher selves.

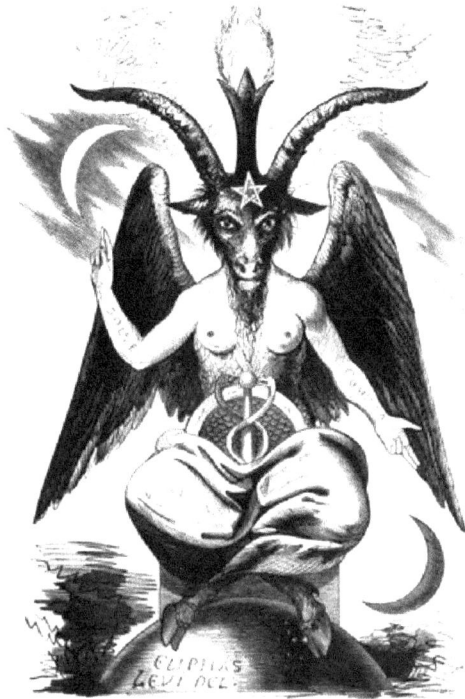

Baphomet oil is suitable for use all year round but its qualities will be especially felt on the winter solstice and full moon. Its essence will resonate strongly with your higher vibrations on these days. The blended oils are designed as an opening portal to awaken the powers of shapeshifting and psychic dreams. It will invoke a sense of being one with nature and promote the feeling of well-being, passion and love. The second night of the full moon (Kapalini) is the night when Baphomet oil acts as a psychopomp, a sublime vessel of transformation.

Using Baphomet perfume oil on the Winter Solstice or Kapalini's nights will help us surrender and let go of old attachments that bind us and prevent us from moving forward.

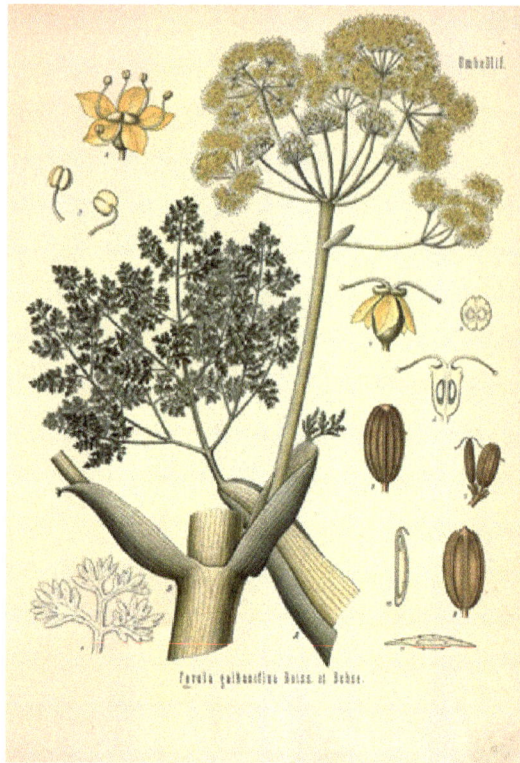

Galbanum, Ferula galbaniflua

(Photo courtesy of wiki commons wikimedia.org)

Galbanum, a large perennial herb belonging to the Umbelliferae family, can be found in the Middle East and Western Asia. It is characterised by its smooth stem and small flowers, as well as resin ducts that give off a natural oleoresin. This is used to derive its Essential oil through either water or steam distillation from the gum.

The potent aroma of Galbanum essential oil encourages dream-filled sleep, evoking memories of decayed timber and freshly unearthed roots. To take it in more mindfully, instils a sensation of being deep underground, perhaps within the ancient pyramids or Paris catacombs.

Galbanum oil had a history of being associated with the mystic and ritualistic. The Egyptians incorporated it into their embalming process and cosmetic formulas, while Romans and Egyptians also used it as incense in their temples and altars. It was even mentioned in the Bible as one of the sweet spices burnt in the Temple at Jerusalem. The potent aroma of the oil brings our minds back to our physical selves and makes us conscious that we need to pass through death in order to reach transformation. Embarking on our olfactory journey, we take the first step with Galbanum. It'll take us into a profound psychic exploration.

In addition to the Galbanum's earthy aroma, we can also sense a warm and spicy fragrance of Opoponax.

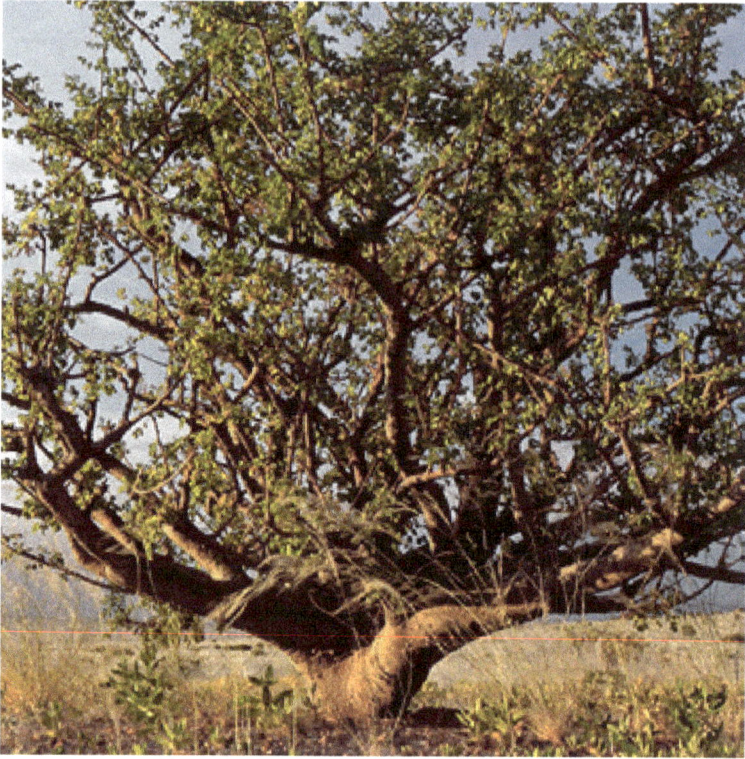

Opoponax, Commiphora erythraea

(Photo courtesy of wiki commons wikimedia.org)

Opoponax is a tall tree, related to Myrrh. It contains a natural oleo gum resin. The gum resin dries and forms tear-shaped lumps of a dark brownish colour. Native to East Africa and extracted from the crude oleo gum resin in two ways:

1.   Essential oil by steam or water distillation.

2.   A resinoid by solvent extraction.

Once the essence of Opoponax oil was discovered, our transformation voyage changed to an enchanted exploration. Its aroma will bring us along a course of self-initiation and enable us to gather our strength for progression. Opoponax oil has long held connections to shapeshifting and enchantment, which can support restoring our spiritual harmony. It carries the influence of all five elements as well as the understanding of intuition.

On each inhalation of Baphomet perfume oil, our olfactory receptors are inundated with the mixture of its scents. After becoming familiar with the base notes of the fragrance, we can detect the fresh and heady, balsamic-spicy aroma emanating from Elemi.

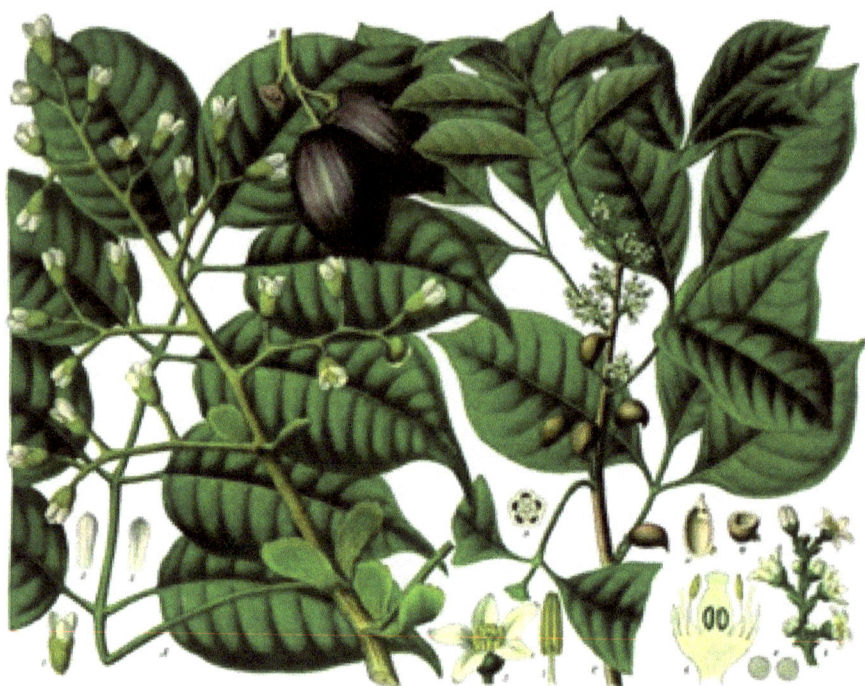

Elemi, Canarium luzonicum

(Photo courtesy of wiki commons wikimedia.org)

Elemi is a tall tropical tree in the Burseraceae botanical group. It originates from the Philippines and Moluccas, known for yielding a resinous gum made up of resin and essential oil. The oil is extracted through steam distillation from the gum.

The smell of Elemi is reminiscent of Frankincense and they both exhibit similar qualities; however, while Frankincense has attained the status of one of the top oils employed by temples and their esteemed priests; like Galbanum, it is believed that Elemi was likely used in embalming practices.

Through my experience with essential oils, I have noticed that the same oils are employed for embalming as well as transformation rituals and rites of passage. Most of them bear the mark of Anubis who is the Master of Secrets and facilitator between realms. When contemplating a meditative state, Frankincense and Elemi alike can help bring you there. Frankincense has a more religious bent to it while Elemi may lead you on a more surreal, psychedelic vision quest. In my imagination, Frankincense is akin to the High Priest of the Temple whereas Elemi feels like Joseph donning his spectacular multi-coloured cloak.

The warm, spicy, sweet honey-like aroma of Elemi resembles the signature note of Frankincense. The deep heady scent of the oil washes our consciousness in a wave of letting go and acceptance and opening our hearts to surrender to the transition, releasing our bonds with the past and moving forward to our next stage of transformation.

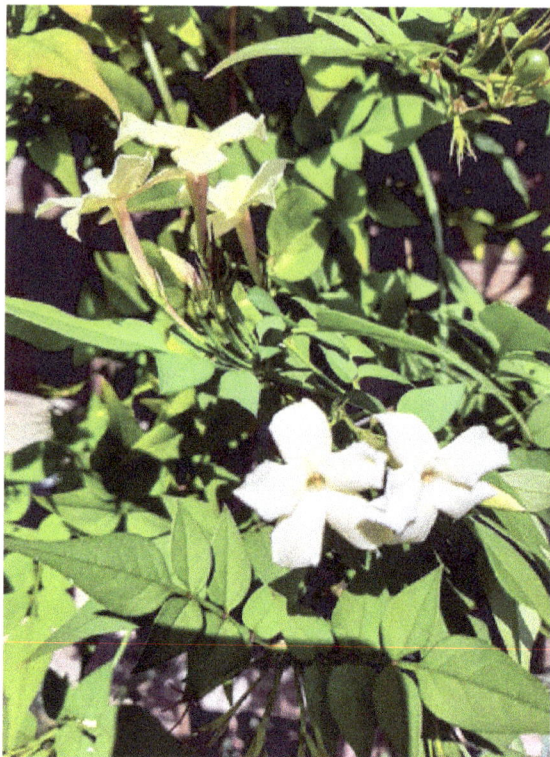

Jasmine, Jasminum officinale

(Photo by the author)

Jasmin is a flowering evergreen shrub that typically reaches heights of 10 metres. A member of the Oleaceae botanical family, it has delicate, bright green leaves and star-shaped flowers that are highly aromatic, ranging from white to yellow in colour. This species is native to China, northern India and western Asia. Its absolute oil is extracted through the enfleurage process whilst its essential oil is derived via steam distillation from the absolute.

Definition: The most concentrated type of fragrance is known as an absolute. It's important to note that absolutes are distinct from essential oils because they contain more than just the oil itself. They also have a higher concentration of plant constituents such as colouring and waxes.

The intense, warm, sweet floral fragrance is immensely powerful in affecting our emotions and can impart a sensation of optimism, assurance and elation. Jasmine is known to act as a sexual stimulant and aphrodisiac and is used to deal with psychological-sexual challenges in either sex. Jasmine is associated with the moon, however, its elemental characteristics are fire and water. This dual character corresponds directly with Baphomet's caduceus/double helix/kundalini energy which grows and is erected from Hir lingam-yoni centre.

The sweet sensual aroma of Jasmine, delicately complements the earthen and herbal notes of the scent, engendering a sense of serenity as it relaxes the body whilst inspiring spiritual awareness, intuition, creative thinking and inventive ideas.

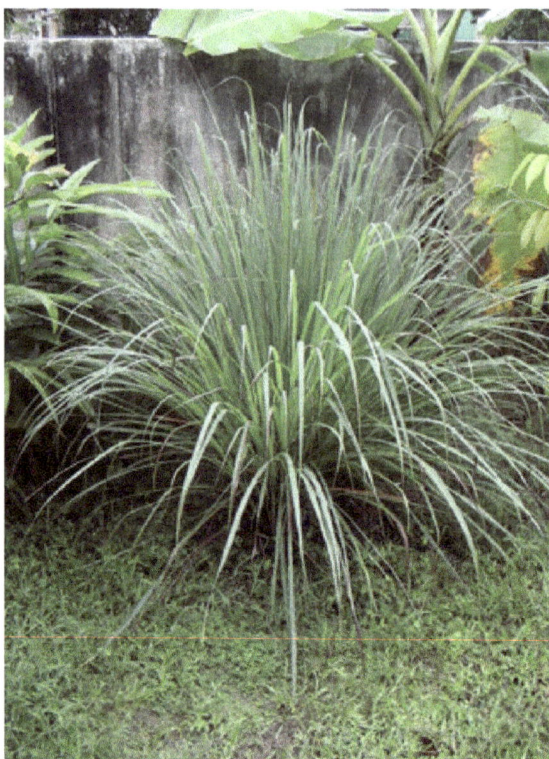

Lemongrass, Cymbopogon citratus

(Photo courtesy of wiki commons wikimedia.org)

Lemongrass is a fast-growing, aromatic perennial tall grass from the Poaceae (Gramineae) botanical family. It is native to Asia. The Essential oil is extracted by steam distillation from the finely chopped fresh and partially dried leaves.

Lemongrass is affiliated with the air element, and its refreshing lemon-herbaceous aroma can be quite compelling. It may bring to mind past visions and fragments of deep and long-lost memories of ancient and untouched wildlands.

Its powerful fragrance stimulates and awakens our psychic mind and purifies our body. The characteristics of Lemongrass

oil combined with the other oils make Baphomet Perfume oil a powerfully transformative, mind-altering, thoughts provoking and insights-inducing initiation oil.

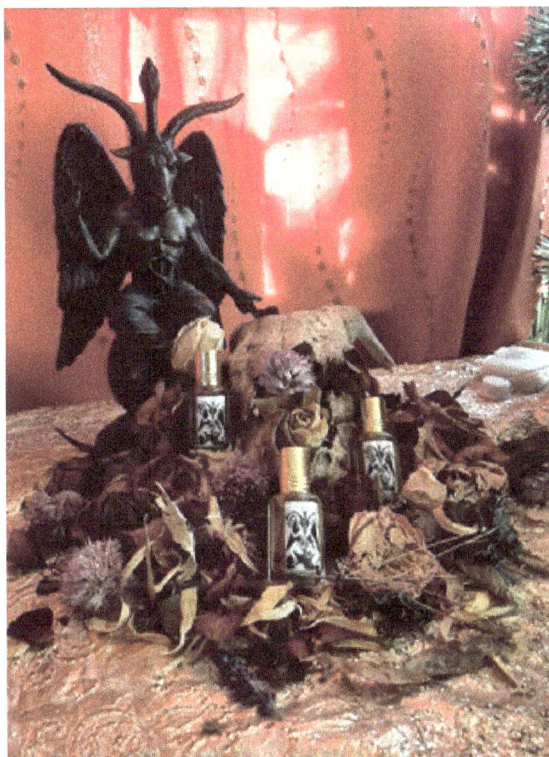

Io Baphomet

This year (2022) marks the perfect union of Mudra Kala and the Winter Solstice. A few nights prior to the new moon, we meet with Mudra Kala, when darkness is profound and the moon is hardly visible, if at all. The Winter Solstice brings along with it the longest night of the year, creating an opportunity for us to delve into our inner emptiness and look for enlightenment through integration with our darkness, the alien and the strange, a true demonic integration (Malphas, The Black Ship: 2009).

Mudra

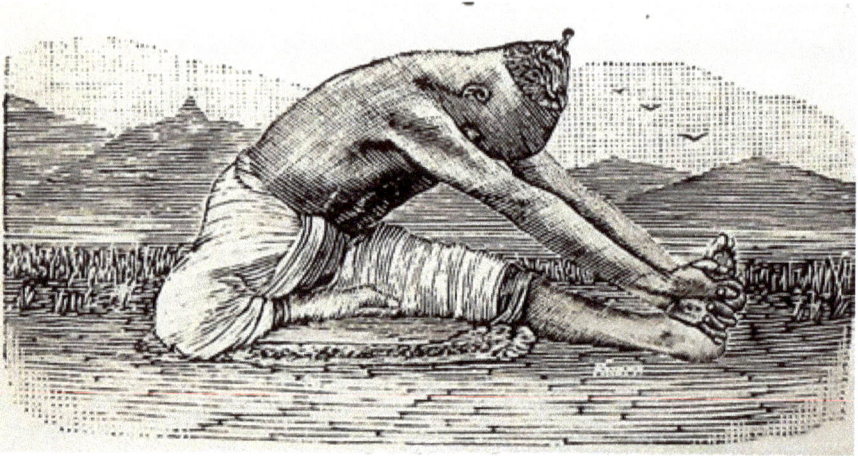

Artist unknown, (Photo courtesy of wiki commons wikimedia.org)

Mudra is the 14th Kala in the Kali sequence. Last night was Mudra night and I was blessed with the most amazing dream:

I was practising the Mahamudra in the foothills of a majestic mountain. As I heard distant Mongolian throat singing, I glanced up and saw Shiva and Buddha radiating with golden light atop the mountain.

> "Mahamudra - the great mudra, is essentially only called this when all three bandhas are involved. The position of the heel in the perineum supports the Mula bandha" (T.K.V Desikachar, *The Heart of Yoga*)

Mahamudra is known as the "great seal" or "great imprint," which reminds us how wisdom and emptiness are inseparably embedded in all aspects of life.

In Vajrayana Buddhism, Mahamudra is the final objective; a union of all dualities. It also has a secret definition as a symbol for 'female partner' who stands for prajna, wisdom or knowledge.

Sometimes the teaching of one dream is worth a lifetime of studies.

12. Green Magick
Imbolc

This chapter is written by my dear friend Miryamdevi, high priestess of the Jitterbug Cult.

To Tom Robbins, Our prophet

* * *

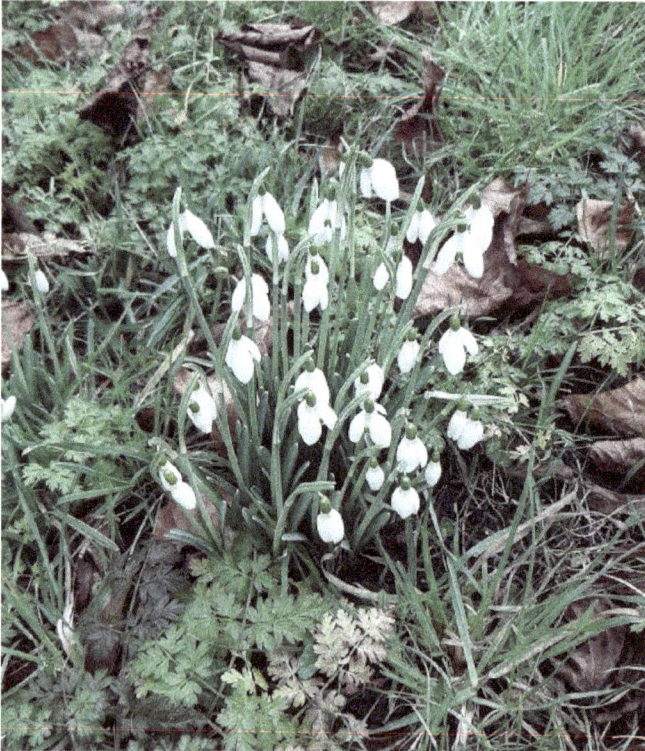

Snowdrops (Photo by the author)

The highest function of Love is that it makes the loved one a unique and irreplaceable being. (Tom Robbins, *Jitterbug Perfume*)

Imbolc marks the midpoint between the winter solstice and spring equinox, a celebration of the world slowly coming back to life. As signs of this, flowers start to reemerge, while buds form on trees. It serves as a reminder that we too can move on from our past, allowing us to make room for fresh starts and new opportunities.

Most snowdrop species blossom in winter, and they are considered to be a symbol of 'hope' and to mark the arrival of spring and the new year.

Green is the colour of nature that speaks to us of growth, stability and

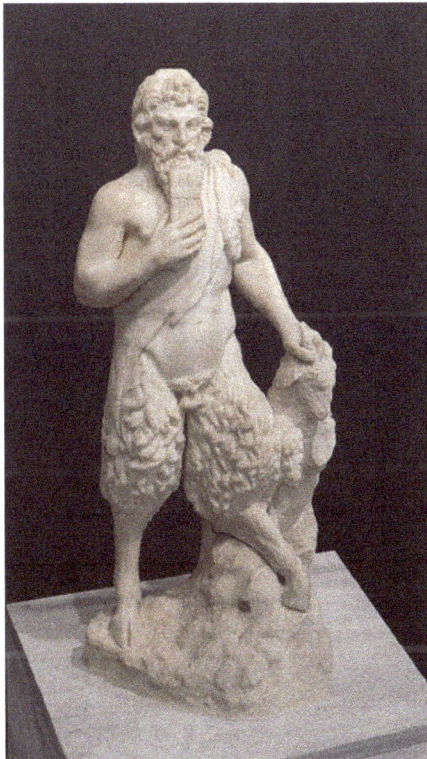

Pan Archmus Heraklion (Photo courtesy of wiki commons wikimedia.org)

resilience. It is an emblem of harmony, healing, fertility, optimism, love and security, inspiring us to open our hearts with enthusiasm for our budding aspirations.

On February first, just before dawn, if you pay close attention, you might just be able to tune in to the entrancing sounds of the panpipes associated with an old god. Furthermore, if you are fortunate enough, you might even catch sight of him doing his peculiar Jitterbug dance as he skips along the shadows.

According to the Greek historian Herodotus, Pan was the most ancient of the gods.

The K23 — Jitterybug Perfume oil

Definition: Essential oils are highly concentrated liquids obtained from plants, containing volatile chemical compounds. These are also known as ethereal oils, volatile oils or simply the oil of the plant from which they were derived.

Definition: Fragrance oils are produced in laboratories to emulate the scents that can be found in nature. There are two main types: synthetic and natural. All of these are artificially created, not directly originating from the environment.

K23 - Ingredients

Grape seed oil & beetroot extract
Horny Goat weed extract

Leather
White Musk
Oud

Amber

Vetiver
Palma Rosa

Jasmine Sambac
Jasmine Officinale
Bergamot
Lemongrass

The above 4 fragrances are representative of the scentual aroma of the body of Pan:

- Leather for flesh and blood.

- White Musk for its earthy, animalistic, sensual qualities like the animal pheromone secretion.

- Oud also known as agarwood is extracted from the fungus-infected resinous heartwood of the Agar tree, which is primarily found in the dense forests of Southeast Asia, India and Bangladesh. It is either extracted by distillation from the wood or by melting the resin. The unique fragrance of Oud is rare and precious, just like the characteristics and charisma of Pan.

- Amber is a 'fantasy' perfumery note. It consists of a few ingredients (natural and synthetic) such as vanilla, patchouli, labdanum, styrax, benzoin and a few more, to create a warm, powdery, sweet scent. The God Pan is the wildest fantasy of mother nature.

The second stage in the manufacture of Jitterybug perfume oil was to replicate a smell that would epitomise the sumptuous, earthy-sharp bouquet of beetroot.

The beetroot is the root part of a Beta vulgaris plant, which has been cultivated for both its edible root and its greens. Beetroots are a great source of many essential vitamins and minerals. It's packed with essential nutrients and is a great source of fibre, folate (vitamin B9), manganese, potassium, iron, and vitamin C and also it contains high concentrations of the element Boron, which is believed to play a key role in producing human sex hormones.

In many cultures, beetroots have been held in high regard as a supposed stimulant of amorous desires.

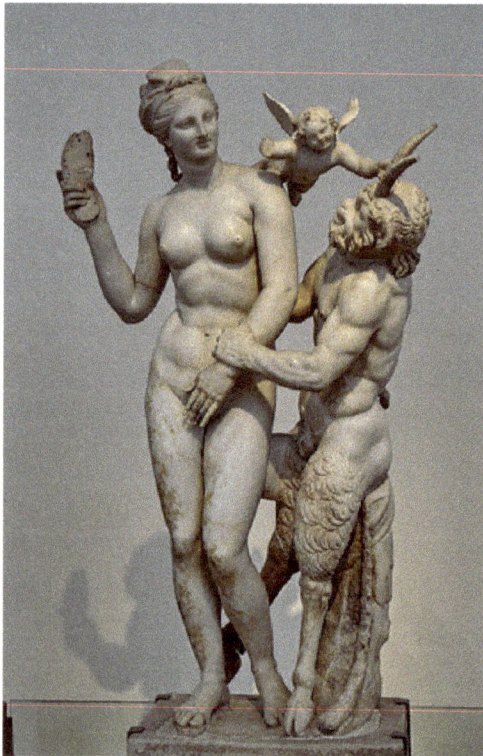

Aphrodite, Eros & Pan, National Archaeological Museum, Athens

(Photo courtesy of wiki commons wikimedia.org)

Aphrodite, the Greek Goddess of Love, Pleasure and Fertility was known and desired for her ageless beauty. Beets were believed to be behind it, and the Oracle at Delphi declared them to be worth their weight in silver due to their enigmatic powers.

In the picture above both God and Goddess seem stimulated after (probably) indulging in just a little too many beets. Poor little Eros appears perplexed – should he join them or intervene?

As previously noted, beetroot is rich in Boron, an element believed to significantly impact the body's production of testosterone and estradiol (a form of estrogen). It seems that both Aphrodite and Pan were well aware of the benefits of the beetroots.

Unfortunately, beetroot doesn't produce any essential oils, so I used a little beet extract as a symbolic gesture. To recreate the scent of the beetroot I used the essential oil of Vetiver and Palmarosa. Vetiver essential oil has a unique smoky, sweet, and earthy-woody aroma like the Earth itself. It brings us closer to our roots in nature through its deep, earthly scent similar to that of beetroot. (For more details about vetiver see the chapter Black Magick).

In his book *Liber Kaos*, Peter Carroll wrote thus on Green Magic: "Invocations to the green power should begin with self-love; an attempt to see the wonderful side of every self one consists of, and then proceed into a ritual affirmation of the beauty and lovability of all things and all people. Suitable god forms for the Love-self include Venus, Aphrodite and the mythical Narcissus…"

In homage to Narcissus, this chapter gives attention to the ancient god of Nature and earth, Pan, who some might declare is gone for good. Nevertheless, he is alive and well in the eyes of the Jitterybug cult - he is the god of Green Magick season.

Io Pan

"Invocations to the green power should begin with self-love"

When we think of self-love, we must take into consideration the differences between Pan and Narcissus. The path of self-love is a narrow one and could lead to destruction through self-delusion, obsession and isolation. This was pretty much Narcissus's way. On the other hand, we have the wild, beasty, earthy way of Pan which can teach us self-love through the appreciation of nature, music and dance. Through pleasures of body, ecstasy and trance, we can learn to see the hidden beauty in every living being and situation. Pan teaches us to have the courage to be wild and leads us to liberation.

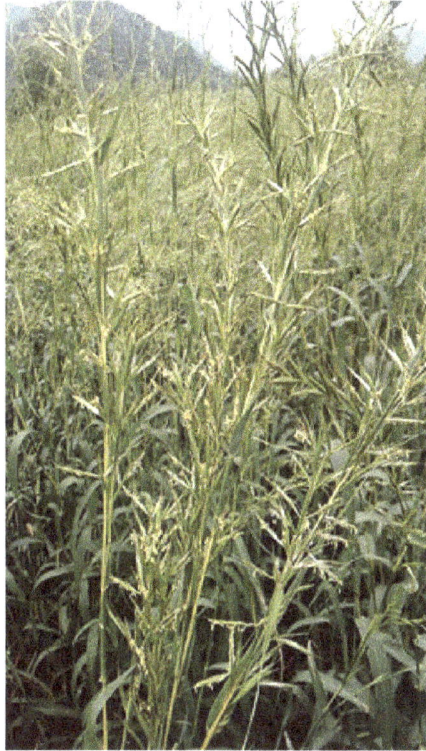

Palmarosa, cymbopogon martinii

(Photo courtesy of wiki commons wikimedia.org)

Palmarosa is an aromatic wild herb that grows in India and Pakistan. It can also be found in Africa, Indonesia, Brazil and the Comoros Islands. The essential oil derived from this plant has a pale yellow or olive hue; it has a sweet, balsamic scent with subtle citrusy and Geranium notes.

While Vetiver is related to the earth element which resonates strongly with Pan and his affinity with the land and nature, Palmarosa is related to the water element which resonates with the flowing nature of love and healing. Both vetiver and palmarosa are under the planetary rule of Venus, which might explain the strange and wild attraction between Pan and Aphrodite in the picture above (Aphrodite, Eros & Pan). The flowing nature of Palmarosa oil soothes the mind and can help heal broken hearts and overcome negative emotions and move forward with our lives.

The Great God Pan is Dead?

In the story, "De Defectu Oraculorum" Plutarch wrote:

> "[the] ship drove with the tide till it was carried near the Isles of Paxi; when immediately a voice was heard … calling unto one Thamus, and that with so loud a voice as made all the company amazed; … the voice said aloud to him, 'When you arrive at Palodes, take care to make it known that the great god Pan is dead.' … this voice did much to astonish all that heard it, and caused much arguing whether this voice was to be obeyed or slighted…"

The news of Pan's passing spread throughout the Roman Empire under Emperor Tiberius' rule. As the realm of antiquity expanded, it took a toll on the natural world, and Pan's existence was no exception. Pan was the God of the Wild and his essence filled his surroundings with life and vitality. Nature was at its most bountiful when Pan was present.

The death of Pan symbolizes the transition from pre-Christian paganism to Christianity and its effect on nature. The expansion of the Roman Empire saw a wave of roads built, leading to an increase in settlements along these paths, disrupting animal and plant species' habitats. Pan's name could also mean 'all', suggesting that his demise may have been the passing of all pre-Christian demons. The goat-legged god became personified as the devil, with his figure appearing in Christian literature and art as the representation of Satan.

However, besides Plutarch's work, there was no indication that Pan had ever died. A century after Plutarch's time, Pausanias described shrines, grottos and sacred caves devoted to Pan that were still very much in use for rituals and pilgrimage.

> In the second aeon, Men knew me as the Horned God, Pangenitor Panphage (Verse 0 Book 1: Sacred scriptures of the Jitterybug cult)

> Pan is not Dead. He is Just resting (Verse 1 Book 1: Sacred scriptures of the Jitterybug cult)

Pan knew that to shake off the satanic image the New Christians imposed on him, he must go into hiding. But as he was the God of nature and a potent emblem of the land, Pan realised they would hunt for him throughout all creation. Those new rulers of the land would track down his trail and detect him from a million miles away. Therefore, he resorted to a different plan; submerging himself in the depths of the sea, where not even his most powerful pheromones could be detected.

Thamus, an Egyptian sailor cruising the Ionian Sea, was startled to hear a mysterious voice proclaim from afar, "The great god Pan is dead!" As he sailed towards Italy, the rumour spread across the Greek islands. Plutarch neglect to mention that Thamus was likely a devout follower of Pan, with some claiming he was one of his most renowned high priests, who may have initiated the tale as a means to maintain the balance and harmony of the land by permitting creatures to stay true to their wilder nature.

The sacred scriptures of the Jitterybug cult tell us how Kudra created a special scent, a perfume to mask the scent of Pan, so he can walk free among us without being detected or recognised, the K23. Kudra had to draw on her expertise in perfumery and understanding of fragrances to mask the pong from Pan. As most of you would be aware, he is the deity in charge of wildernesses, herds and flocks – his half-goat form is quite a distinctive sight. And unless you have been to a shepherd's pen full of goats, it can be hard to imagine how powerful their scent can be! Especially with the males - let's just say they don't smell so great. Creating a perfume suitable for a god is a serious task, even more so if the perfume in mind needs to conceal the scent of one of the odiferous gods around.

Kudra was somewhat vague about the ingredients she used to create the K23. We know she collected the very rare pollen of the beetroot to balance out with earthy tones and the animalistic stench of the goat, and then she added the best quality Jasmine oil she could find. In Kudra's case, it will probably be ok to assume she used Jasmine Sambac.

Jasmine has the honour of being one of the highest-priced plant scents and has often been called the king of flowers. (Scott Cunningham:1997).

Earlier in the book, Jasmine was also dedicated to the Amrita Kala (Amrita means "immortality") and resonates with the sexual magic elixir. It is also associated with Lalita. Lalita is a Hindu goddess, worshipped as a principal aspect of the supreme goddess Mahadevi. The intense scent of Jasmine can affect our emotions by producing feelings of optimism, confidence and euphoria in the hearts of the devotees when worshipping the gods. The powerful aroma of Jasmine will be sufficient to tone down the stench of the goat, and at the same time will support its life essence and vitality, sexual appeal and stamina, which are so vital for the man-goat-God Pan. Kudra suggested that the finishing touch to the perfume should be a light scent from the citrus family, and I thought Bergamot would be ideal. After all, what is better than the fresh, sweet and uplifting brightness of Bergamot to help keep one's energy moving effortlessly throughout the body and mind. However, after letting the blend settle, it became apparent that one final note was required to make it complete.

So what would it be?

I really struggled to choose between the invigorating, herbaceous-lemony aroma of Lemongrass and the equally fresh, zesty-floral scent of Lemon-Verbena. Eventually, I settled on Lemongrass. Octarine Magick's chapter described it perfectly; its intense lemony-herbal scent can evoke long-forgotten memories of untouched wildernesses.

This version of the K23 is an intricate, paradoxical mix of aromas, scents and smells. Writing this chapter was a voyage that guided me through the pulsing Green Magick, something I never could have anticipated when starting my task. It is only with gratitude that I can look upon the author who spotted my ability and familiarity with the ancient rituals of the last God who still knows how to dance the Jitterbug.

Before I go, I entrust you with the cult's most sacred scripture — the teaching of St Beetaroota and the secret of the beets.

February 20k23
Miryamdevi, Jitterbug priestess

St Beetaroota

If there is no St Beetaroota there really ought to be, so here goes.

A few weeks after Imbolc, St. Beetaroota Day is celebrated on February 14th. This commemorates the love affair between Beetaroota and Pan, as well as highlights how the humble winter root is an essential element of two of the most renowned magical formulas in history.

St Beetaroota CE 640 - 666 was St Sexburger's younger half-sister. St Beetaroota was born out of wedlock and unlike her sister, she spent most of her life in a tiny and very poor village in Essex, working the Beet fields.

One day, she was overcome by an intense aroma. She felt her head swooning as she tried to find out its origin, only to discover a handsome man sleeping beside a large boulder located in the middle of the field. She tentatively moved toward him and cried out in surprise. "Oh, what an exquisite goat!" This made him leap to his feet and head in her direction. Its powerful odour was enough to make her faint, sending her flying into the beetroot patch.

Lying on the ground, Beetaroota had a dream. The god Pan manifested before her and offered to share the knowledge of beets with her. Once she awoke and opened her eyes, Pan towered over her with a grin on his face. Instinctively, she reaches for one of the beets and brought it close

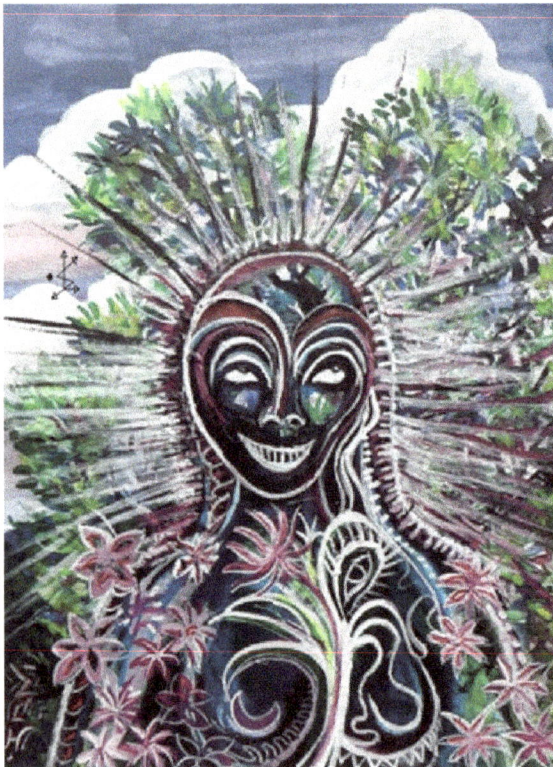

Black Tantric Goddess by Jan Fries, 2019

to her nose, promptly realising that its smell cancelled out the odour of the Man-God-Creature. Pan seated himself on a rock and began playing the most entrancing melody Beetaroota had ever heard. The music spread throughout the area and it was as if a warm mist was emitted from the beet plants; everything around her seemed to move slowly. Butterflies and bees scattered around in the beaming field, with an especially enthralling scent wafting through the air, bringing a smile to Beetaroota's face.

I understand now, she said. Pan took her hand and kissed her.

Remember, he said, the magickal essence can be collected only today and only between sunrise and sunset. This essence will provide you with the most unique ingredient for the invisibility potion, it will musk any offensive smells and unique phenomena. It is also the secret ingredient in the ancient formula of the evocation of me. Please use it with extra caution.

He was gone.

From this day forth, Beetaroot's village was renowned for its abundant supply of the largest, most succulent beets in the nation; supplying even the king with their crop. The modest village swiftly became one of the wealthiest settlements in the area. Beetaroota became a healer, taking advantage of her beets in her medicinal and magical mixtures; people from all corners of the nation sought after her help and blessings.

Every year on the 14th of February, just before dawn, Beetaroota ventured out to her field in search of Pan. Though he never appeared, the field was covered with a magickal warm hazy glow; from this, she harvested ingredients for her healing medicines, perfumes and potions.

On February 14th CE 666, Beetaroota made her way to the field before dawn and was never seen from then on. It was rumoured that she had been spotted exiting the area alongside a being with goat-like features.

Once she went missing, the people of the village adorned a huge boulder from her plot with red paint. Since then, every year on February 14th, offerings of beets and blossoms were placed around it as a mark of respect.

13. Orange Magick
Spring equinox

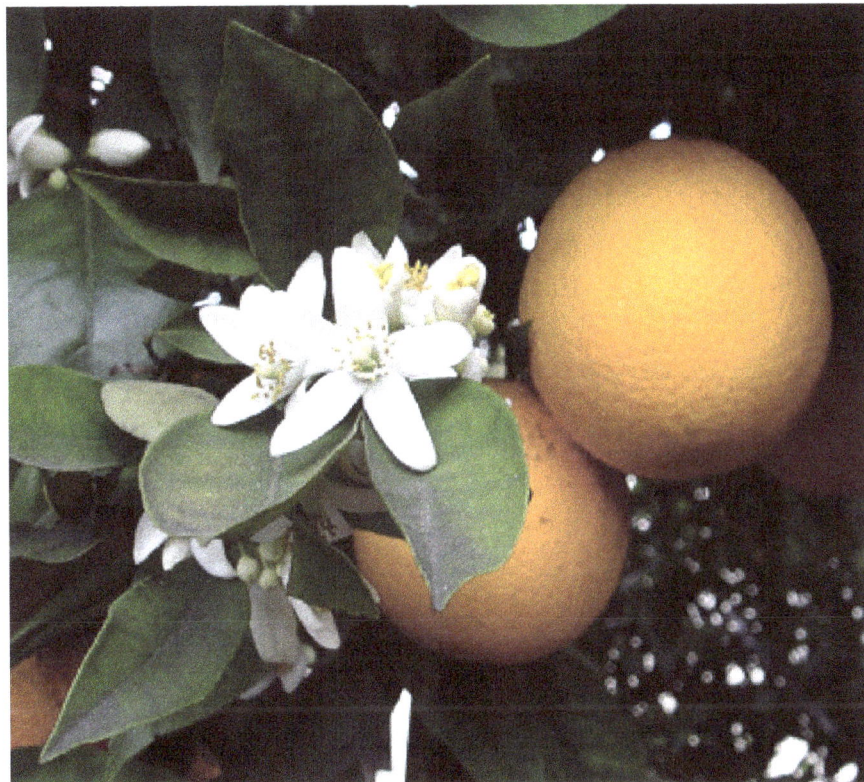

(Photo courtesy of wiki commons wikimedia.org)

Twice a year the wheel stops for a moment when the sun is situated exactly above the equator and day and night are of equal length. This happens on the Spring and Autumn Equinoxes. Now the day and the night are equal, a symbolic representation of our need for balance during this period.

The spring equinox bring with it new beginnings, renewal and growth. According to Chinese lore, orange is the ideal combination of yellow and red – a colour synonymous with spontaneous change, adaptability and transformation. It evokes feelings of success, confidence, delight, brightness and warmth. Not surprisingly, due to its connection with seasonal fluctuations, it can represent change and movement. According to "Orange Magic" in *Liber Kaos* (Peter Carroll: 1992) "Charlatanry, trickery, living by one's wits and thinking fast on one's feet are the essence of the orange power." Reading on, Peter also tells us that "charlatanry still has its place in magic".

> "The antiquated meaning of 'glamour' is witchcraft. The most important asset to the modern witch is her ability to be alluring, to utilize glamour. The word 'fascination' has a similarly occult origin." (Anton LaVey)

Glamour, fascination, conjure, sleight of hands, hypnotism, mesmerism, illusions, psychological manipulation, all of this could be understood as charlatanry, or, magic. Anton LaVey referred to this type of art as 'Lesser Magic'.

Lesser magic is the art of manipulating psychology to achieve desired results. It involves adapting techniques depending on the context, whether that be an interview, a conversation with a child, addressing a group or negotiating with authorities. With practice, one can gain mastery over various intimidating and disheartening situations.

Orange magic aids us in attaining equilibrium between the tranquil and clear energy of yellow magic and the vigorous force of red magic. To reach peak performance with yellow and red magic, fascination and glamour techniques should be employed by the magician through the use of orange magic.

The sweet and citrusy fragrance of the orange has an immediate effect on us, transforming our mood and lifting our spirits. It opens our hearts, filling them with joy and cleansing our aura. According to Gabriel Mojay's *Aromatherapy for Healing the Spirit*, the principal value of the orange, "lies in its ability to unblock and circulate stagnant Qi-energy". The orange essence has a special ability, which can be likened to how a magician might employ minor magic techniques like unblocking an area or promoting energy flow. Additionally, this power can be employed to read hidden messages, create protective charms, perform ceremonies, invocations or banishing.

The Bitter orange tree (Citrus aurantium var. amara) is an evergreen with a smooth, greyish trunk and branches. Dark green, glossy leaves and very fragrant white flowers adorn the tree which can reach up to 10 metres high. Its fruit, smaller and darker than the sweet orange, is believed to be the ancestor of all existing varieties of Citrus plants. It is native to the Far East yet also thrives in areas such as the Mediterranean, California, Israel and South America.

> "If we think in trinities, things will flow more."
> (Lionel Snell, TransStates Conference 2022)

The age-old secret of the sacred trinity is encased within the essence of a tree. This olfactory riddle is only known to those versed in perfume and aromatherapy. Like an illusionist conjuring a rabbit out of thin air, the unassuming bitter orange tree with its unpalatable fruits contains a holistic trio of enchanting aromas. Before sharing this mystery, let us consider the symbolism behind the number three.

The ancient Egyptian religion is known for its frequent use of divine triads, which appear in many places. Each city had its own divine triad and the most famous one is the Abydos triad — Osiris, Isis and Horus. Some of the more well-known triads you will find in Edfu - Horus, Hathor and Harsomtus, Memphis – Ptah, Sekhmet and Nefertum, Heliopolis -

Khepri-Re-Atum, Karnak – Amun, Mut and Khonsu.

Edfu Temple, located in southern Egypt and dedicated to the god Horus, is the second largest surviving temple in the country. Covering its walls are various inscriptions known as the Edfu Texts, which include recipes of sacred perfumes and incense used in daily rituals. Dora Goldsmith, an Egyptologist, translated some of these recipes and teaches about them in her distinctive workshops and classes. Once I began constructing the Ti-Sps — Hathor's sacred perfume oil — the trilateral divisions were evident in all the passions of ancient Egyptians. Crafting the Ti-Sps was ruled by threefold mysticism, a process that stretched over 243 days, an endeavour you can learn more about in a future book of the Aromagick series.

Three is the smallest number we need to create a pattern. It's a principle captured neatly in the Latin phrase omne trium perfectum: everything that comes in threes is perfect, or, complete. It was considered to be the perfect number, the number of harmony, wisdom and understanding.

It represents the three different timelines:

Past, present, future
Birth, life, death
Beginning, middle, end
The number three, was the number of the divine.

In the pursuit of the divine scent, the one that will unlock our souls and bring forward the illuminating wisdom of our inner mind, we overlooked and disregarded the unassuming Bitter Orange tree. As I wrote earlier, the tree hides within its branches a holistic triad of essential oils: Orange, Neroli (Orange blossom) and Petitgrain.

When we squeeze the peel of the orange fruit, it releases a sweet citrusy warm aroma which will immediately lift our hearts with transformative energy, promoting happiness and peace. The scent of the Orange oil promotes magical energy and can be used to banish negative thoughts, jealousy and insecurities. Its principal value, to unblock and circulate stagnant energy, can be woven into spells for harmonising and balancing relationships, prosperity and good fortune.

Growing up on a farm engulfed by Orange groves, I will never forget the captivating scent of the blossoms. The mild autumn breeze made my walks with the farm dogs an aromatic extravaganza, and the strong smell of Neroli, wafting on the delicate autumn winds, felt like a cleansing ritual of aromas that invigorated and cheered me up. It seemed like even the dogs were enjoying it, their joyful tails endlessly wagging, their playful behaviour.

Neroli has a luxurious and heady scent that generates magical effects, purifying the mind of any mental negativity and heavy emotions. Its paradoxical intensity of lightness will help one's stress dissipate, bring a smile to your face and even cause a sense of euphoria. For centuries, orange blossoms have been highly sought-after for their ability to bring peace and balance to the mind and the heart. They have been particularly popular in bridal wreaths and headdresses.

In the past, the oil of Petitgrain was extracted from the small green unripe oranges – hence the name petitgrain or 'little grains'. Today the oil is produced only from the leaves and twigs of the same tree that produces Bitter Orange and Orange blossom oil. The fresh green aroma of Petitgrain is closely reminiscent of orange blossom, yet in contrast to the calming scent of the flower, Petitgrain presents a sharp and invigorating aroma. Working with it reinforces its refreshing and energising nature, as well as acquainting you with the whole tree's under and overtones. The sharpness of its smell will awaken your senses and fill you with vitality.

The Orange, Neroli and Petitgrain are ruled by the Sun and correspond to the element of fire. This is echoed in the harmony produced by the Bitter Orange tree reflecting the balance of solar energies during the spring equinox. The Sun has long been prized for its power to protect and bring life, cheer and delight, a reminder of the special properties infused into each of these essential oils.

14. Purple Magick
Mayday/Beltane

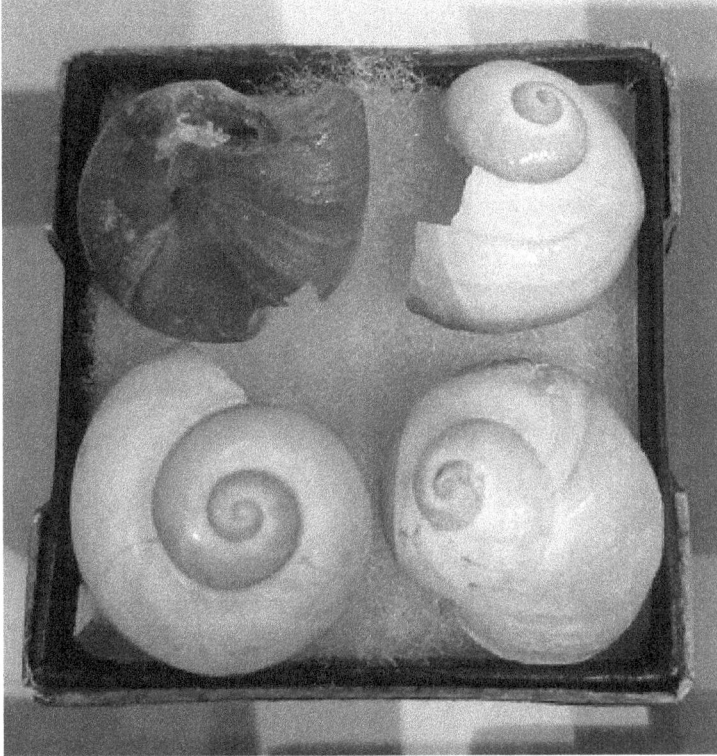

(Photo by the author, Pitt Rivers Museum, Various collections)

These sea snail shells were excavated from Roman sites near Tyre in Lebanon. The creatures inside were crushed and boiled in a salt solution to produce the famous 'Tyrian Purple'. It took 10,000 snails to produce just 1.4 grams of dye, making it very valuable and it became the preserve of Emperors, hence its alternative name, 'imperial purple'. (Pitt Rivers Museum, Various collections)

The rites of Mayday, or Beltane, are celebrated between the spring equinox and the summer solstice in the northern hemisphere. This tradition is believed to have been celebrated since antiquity. Across Europe, festivities on May 1st usually involve dancing around a decorated Maypole - a phallic symbol adorned with floral garlands representing blooming fertility and sexual vigour. Beltane is an important festival in Gaelic culture, alongside Samhain, Imbolc, and Lughnasadh. It was once widely celebrated in Ireland, Scotland, and the Isle of Man. The occasion centred around ritualistic bonfires that were believed to possess protective powers. People and animals would encircle or even jump through these blazing fires. On this day, all domestic fires were extinguished and relit from the Beltane bonfire.

I've always been drawn to the colour purple. It brings together the serenity of blue and the vibrancy of red, inspiring me to express my emotions. Purple triggers my imagination and encourages me to explore new ideas. Purple encourages spiritual advancement and promotes comprehension and tolerance. It reminds me that there are a wealth of amazing mysteries out there to be discovered. Yet, even as I explore them, purple keeps me rooted and prompts me to stay attuned to what really matters in life.

> "4. The deep violet is episcopal. It combines 2 and 3, a bishop being the manifestation of heavenly or starry existence manifested through the principle of blood or animal life." (Column XV, King Scale of Colour, *The Qabalah of Aleister Crowley*).

The colour purple is like a bishop when it comes to colours. It is formed by combining the red of blood and the blue of the sky, allowing us to explore an array of complex feelings. Red embodies blood, fire, love, passion, warmth, lust and sexuality along with blue signifying the sky, freedom, intuition, imagination, inspiration and depth. This brilliant blend provides us with balance and abundance while simultaneously granting us liberty to be inspired by our own sexuality, ardour, desire and creativity.

"The colour violet, generally speaking, signifies a vibration which is at the same time spiritual and erotic; i.e. it is the most intense of the vibrations alike on the planes of Nephesch and Neschamah…" (Column XV, The Zodiacal Attributions: *The Qabalah of Aleister Crowley*)

Using a variety of aliases, Crowley was often referred to as the Beast 666 and Count von Zonaref, in addition to Alastair McGregor. Moreover, he sometimes employed "The Purple Priest" as a pseudonym to demonstrate his authority within the church of Thelema. This title is associated with certain high-ranking roles in the clergy, including that of a bishop or senior bishop. Crowley employs purple as an erotically-spiritual symbol throughout Thelema's rituals and worship, conveying a deeper, esoteric meaning.

In *Liber Al – The Book of the Law*, 1:61, we can see how Crowley uses the colour purple in his writings:

"But to love me is better than all things: if under the night stars in the desert thou presently burnest mine incense before me, invoking me with a pure heart, and the Serpent flame therein, thou shalt come a little to lie in my bosom. For one kiss wilt thou then be willing to give all; but whoso gives one particle of dust shall lose all in that hour. Ye shall gather goods and store of women and spices; ye shall wear rich jewels; ye shall exceed the nations of the earth in splendour & pride; but always in the love of me, and so shall ye come to my joy. I charge you earnestly to come before me in a single robe, and covered with a rich headdress. I love you! I yearn to you! Pale or purple, veiled or voluptuous, I who am all pleasure and purple, and drunkenness of the innermost sense, desire you. Put on the wings, and arouse the coiled splendour within you: come unto me!"

By using metaphors such as pale or purple, the author might be hinting at the physiology of the lingam. "Pale" suggests a flaccid lingam, and "veiled" could be the stage just before the lingam is fully erect, also it might suggest an uncircumcised lingam. "Purple" suggests its "voluptuous" erection. There are several veins and arteries that carry blood to and from the spongy erectile tissue in the penis. Veins may look larger than usual during and immediately following an erection. The appearance of prominent veins indicates healthy blood flow and gives the lingam a purple hue.

Next, the colour purple is used to describe the Priestess-Goddess, Nuit: "I who am all pleasure and purple" — here purple is used as a metaphor for the yoni — the purple pleasure … By using those metaphors, the purple priest emphasises the intensity and depth of the spiritual and erotic vibration in religious-like practices of carnal pleasures. The second half of the sentence - "and drunkenness of the innermost sense," hints at the ecstatic heights of the orgasm that awaits in the palace (Liber Al 1:51). The Palace is another metaphor for the yoni - see Mogg Morgan's *Aleister Crowley & Thelemic Magick* page 39.

In his "Hymn to Pan" we can see the "purple motif" again:

> "…Dip the purple of passionate prayer
> In the crimson shrine, the scarlet snare,
> The soul that startles in eyes of blue
> To watch thy wantonness weeping through…"

There is something very special at this time of the year, the ancient earth dragon, Kundalini, is now fully awakened. The air is fragrant with the sweet heady aromas of many colourful blossoms. Insects, animals and humans alike walk or crawl out of their burrows, rub their eyes, stretch their limbs and start dancing a sensual mating dance. It's the season to celebrate desire, lust, fertility, or in other words, nature's tantric celebration.

This is the season of Pan, the "All-devourer, all-begetter". There is something very salacious about dancing around a Maypole. And by leaping over the Beltane fires, we awaken the most ancient magick of all, the passion for the union of body and spirit — "a vibration which is at the same time spiritual and erotic".

This is the perfect time to wear the K23 perfume oil which will connect you to the spirit of Pan and his passionate lust for earth and life. Then, go outside and do the Jitterbug.

The term jitterbug is used to refer to different swing dances, such as the jive and the lindy hop. It comes from slang used in the early twentieth century to describe alcoholics. The term became associated with swing dancers because, like the jitters of alcoholics, they were seen to be out of control.

As discussed earlier in the book, the properties of water allow us spiritual cleansing, where immersion in a ritual bath is always desirable and recommended before magical activity. To connect with the purple magic frequency and awaken the energies of the Kundalini serpent I recommend my special purple bath ritual which is specifically designed to raise our sexual and magnetic powers and to synchronise ourselves with potential or existing partners. Partners can share their bath in the spirit of a purple magick ritual for play, however, here at the Morgan Witches' headquarters, we prefer to have our ritual baths separately (usually one after the other) and by doing so, each of us has the time to relax and meditate. It takes 15 minutes for our body to reach a general relaxation that allows the blend of oils to work its magick on our consciousness.

Prepare your bathroom as you would any other ritual space, you can have a 'purple altar' if you have the room for it, but remember that the altar is the bath, and the water is the vessel which conducts the transformation of the offering which in this case is the oils and you. When using the Purple Magick Perfume Oil you can add about 10-15 drops to a tablespoon of sea salt, Himalayan salt or Epsom salts and add it to the bath water. Each of the essential oils suggested here can be used on its own or in combination with one of the other essential oils which are recommended in this chapter. However, mixing and blending essential oils is a form of art and technique that need to be learned and mastered. You can use the recipe at the end of the chapter as a guideline for making your own bath blends.

Ensure that the water is sufficiently warm to allow you to relax for 15 minutes. Lie in the water comfortably, close your eyes, take a few deep breaths and tune into the mantra or music you love.

I find that the Kirtan Kriya (Sa Ta Na Ma) mantra is most suitable to listen to in the purple bath ritual.

You can find it here: youtube.com/watch?v=NNwAz2BRsak.

If you want to experience the purple magick in its full power I recommend the Great Purple Hoo-Ha meditation while in the bath. The Kirtan Kriya mantra will amplify the experience.

The Great Purple Hoo-Ha Meditation

This meditation is based on a technique described in the book The Great Purple Hoo-Ha by Phillip H. Farber, an esteemed writer, hypnotist, NLP trainer, ritualist and consciousness explorer. Farber's notable works include Future Ritual: Magick for the 21st Century and he is the originator of Meta-Magick - a practice which fuses magick, NLP, hypnosis and more.

Sit in a comfortable position with your spine upright (if you are in the bath, just make yourself comfortable and relax in the water). Close your eyes.

Imagine a circle around you, with a diameter just slightly greater than your outstretched arms, with you at the exact centre.

Inhale, filling your lungs completely, from bottom to top.

As you inhale, allow your attention to expand and fill the circle around you with purple.

Exhale, and as you do so place your attention to a tiny spot within the centre of your chest.

Continue to practice like this, filling the circle with every inhalation, contracting down to a single point in the middle of your chest. When your circle is full of purple, inhale and expand your attention to fill the entire room with purple.

Then, when you exhale, contract it down to a single point in the centre of your chest.

Once the room is full of purple, on the next inhalation expand your attention to fill the largest area you can conceive: the city, the county, the state, the world or even the solar system and the whole universe, with the colour purple. As large as you can manage. And again, when you exhale, contract your attention down to a single point in the middle of your chest.

When you are ready, open your eyes and return to your regular breathing. Thank yourself, the water and the oils, climb out of the bath, dry yourself and get dressed (or not) and carry on with your Purple Magick celebrations.

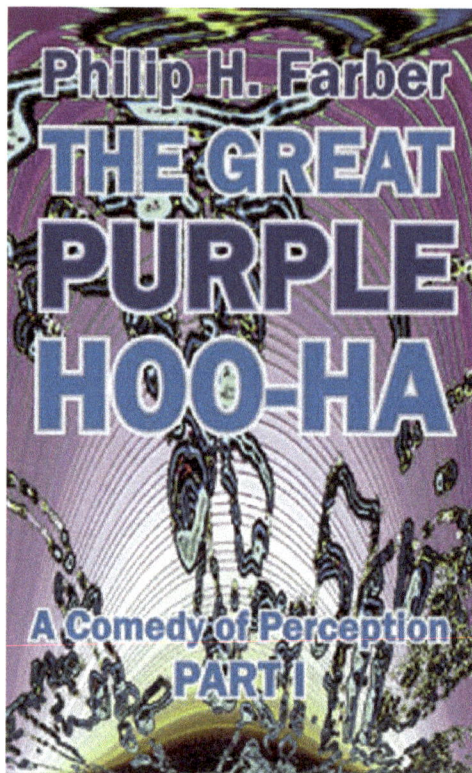

Philip H. Farber
THE GREAT
PURPLE
HOO-HA
A Comedy of Perception
PART I

Purple Magick Perfume Oil

The first essential oil that comes to mind concerning Purple Magick, as Scott Cunningham put it "downtrodden Patchouli". Even now, most people still associate its sweet musky and earthy aroma with the 'Hippy' culture of the 1960s & 70s.

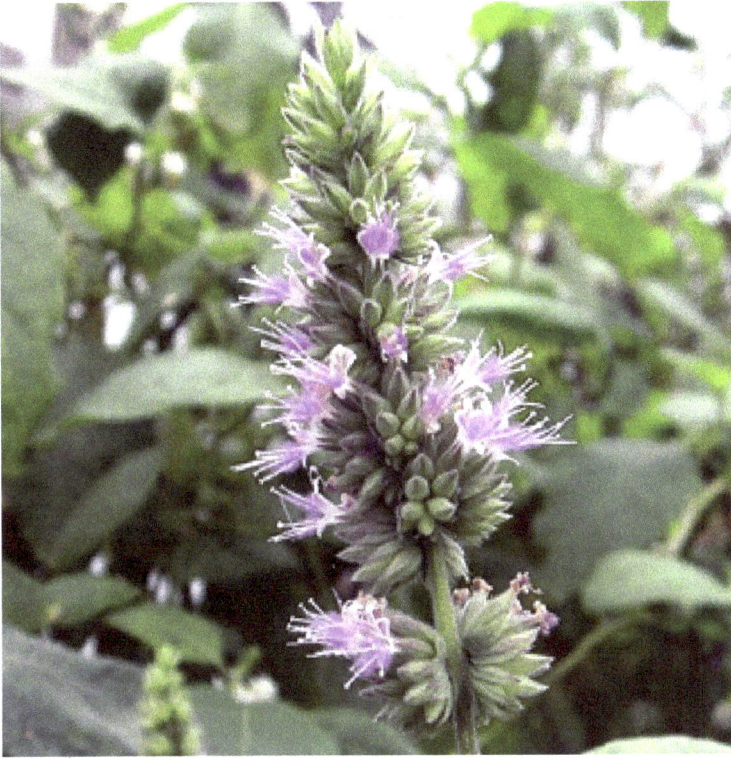

Patchouli, Pogostemon cablin

(Photo courtesy of wiki commons wikimedia.org)

Patchouli is a bushy herb, native to Southeast Asia and grows to a height of one metre. It has a sturdy, hairy stem and large, fragrant leaves that are furry to touch. The white-purple flowers bloom in the summer. After harvesting the patchouli leaves, they're left in the shade for fermentation which gives the oil high quality when extracted through steam distillation after three days of drying.

In the 19th century, cashmere shawls and bed linen were imported from India to Europe. To keep the delicate fabrics free of moths, they were packed with patchouli leaves, which were used throughout the East as an insect repellent. These Patchouli-scented shawls and linen became a must-have item for well-to-do and fashionable women of the time. It didn't

take long for the Patchouli fragrance to be associated with wealth and indulgence.

The distinctive sweet earthiness of Patchouli soon became a popular trait amongst European fabric and furniture producers, who began to incorporate the scent into their products. This conjures up visions of luxurious, musky bedrooms in the 19th century that were sure to have been fragrant with the aroma. For centuries, the aroma has been thought of as an aphrodisiac. The earthy-musky notes bring about a sense of security and invite relaxation, and provide us with encouragement to explore our own sensuality. The aroma of patchouli oil pervading bed linen and furniture was powerfully evocative and gave those 19th-century bedrooms a sense of seductiveness that has never left our collective memory. So next time you watch a period drama or read a novel set in this era, enhance your experience by having some Patchouli around. Whenever a bedroom scene arises or when a cashmere shawl appears, take the time to smell the scent and really feel involved with the story.

The sweet and heady scent of the Patchouli blends perfectly with the exotic fragrance of Ylang-Ylang. On its own, I find Ylang-Ylang a bit overpowering and far too sweet, but the earthiness of Patchouli seems to anchor the sweetness of the Cananaga odorata and turn it into a somewhat lighter and mysterious exotic fragrance.

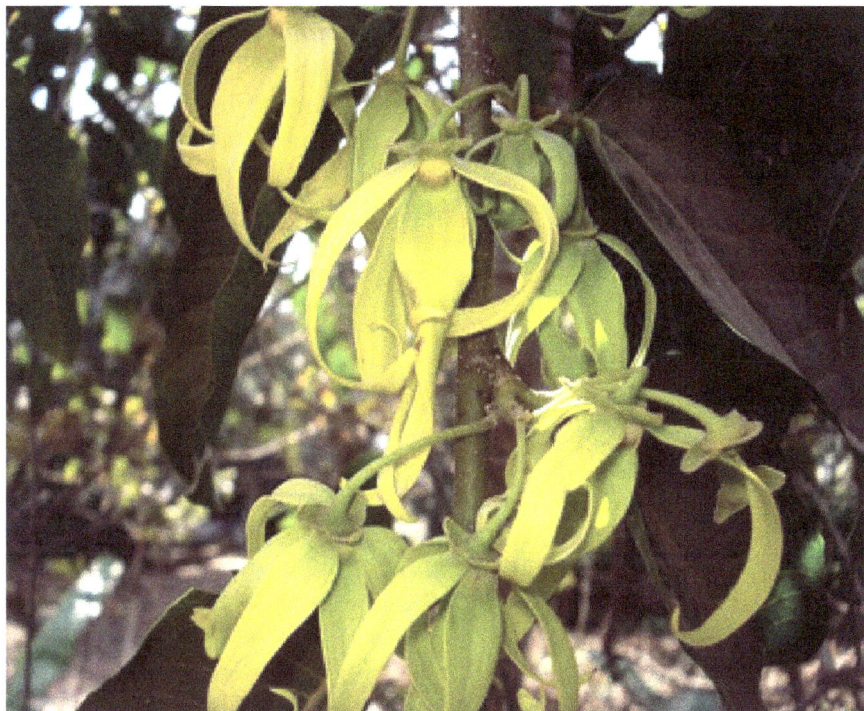

Ylang-Ylang, Cananaga odorata

(Photo courtesy of wiki commons wikimedia.org)

Ylang-Ylang is a tall tropical tree with large, tender, sweet fragrant yellow flowers. It is native to Southeast Asia. Its essential oil is extracted by water or steam distillation from freshly picked flowers. There are 5 grades of distilled essential oil, with Ylang-Ylang extra as the top grade.

The exotic, balsamic aroma of Ylang-Ylang is believed to be an effective balancer and soother for an overactive mind or heightened emotional state. In Indonesia, the flower has long been connected with aphrodisiacs and can be used to create a tranquil yet stimulating atmosphere. On their wedding night, newlyweds often decorate their bed with freshly picked blooms. Both Ylang-Ylang and Vetiver are under the planetary influence of Venus, the goddess of love, beauty and sensuality. Together they combine two of her most precious elements, the stability of the earth represented by Vetiver and the fluidity of water represented by Ylang-Ylang. On the emotional, physiological and magical level, these two oils blended together act as the psychic lubricant of body and mind. Once the harmony between these two Venusian oils has been established, we can introduce Jasmine, the "King of flowers" to the formula (Cunningham: 1997).

Jasmine is known for its qualities as a sexual tonic and aphrodisiac. The intensely rich, warm and sensual, sweet floral scent, has a direct effect on our emotions and can produce a feeling of optimism, confidence and euphoria. Its association with the moon will add a silvery reflection to a sensuous magical rite, where there is a union of lovers. Its elemental characteristics of both fire and water will intensify the sacred sexual union with a magical oomph of flowing passion.

To balance out the richness of the sweet and heady aroma of the blend I added a few drops of Bergamot. The fresh and fruity, citrusy scent of the oil, is just sharp enough to break the nearly overwhelming sweetness of the heady blend.

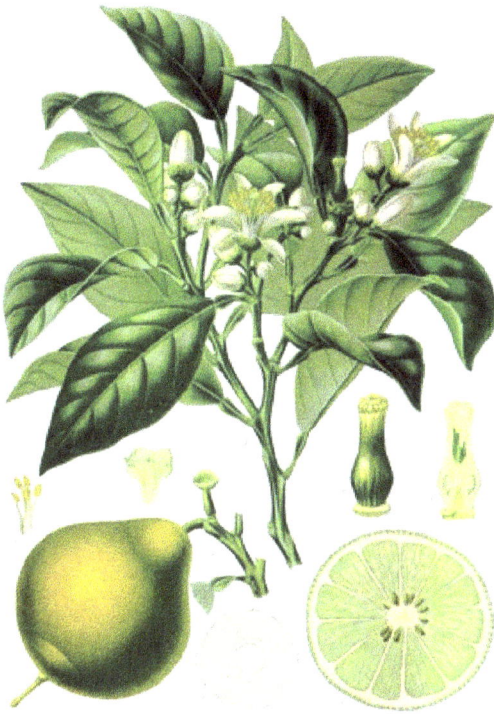

Bergamot, Citrus bergamia

(Photo courtesy of wiki commons wikimedia.org)

This small tree, about 4.5 metres high with smooth oval leaves, and small round fruit, ripens from green to yellow, similar to orange in appearance but smaller. Native to tropical Asia. Extensively cultivated in southern Italy, Sicily and the Ivory Coast. Essential oil extraction is by cold expression of the fruit's rind.

Safety data: Certain furocoumarins, notably bergapten, are phototoxic on human skin; that is, they cause sensitisation and skin pigmentation when exposed to direct sunlight.

The scent of Bergamot resembles that of orange but with more floral and zesty underlying characteristics that add a spicy edge to it. Bergamot possesses magical qualities that can alleviate nervous tension and physical stress, acting like a wand by lifting, shifting, releasing, and dispersing these feelings. Bringing peace and happiness and creating a space allows both body and mind to rest and relax. The lightness and uplifting touch that Bergamot adds to the blend, accentuates each of the other fragrances and mixes them into a bewitching sensual perfume which will work both ways on its wearer and their partner.

Purple Magick bath recipe:

In a small bowl, mix 1 tablespoon of sea salt, Himalaya salt or Epsom salt,

1 drop of Patchouli

1 drop Ylang Ylang

2 drops of Jasmine

3 drops of Bergamot

For your safety, I recommend using the following recipe for a night-time bath due to the sensual nature of purple magick and the potential risks associated with Bergamot essential oil.

It's important to note that the Purple Magic Perfume Oil is safe to use as it contains bergaptene-free essential oil.

15. Yellow Magick
Summer Solstice

And here we are, once again, at that time of the year when a unique portal opens up. As the summer solstice approaches, we catch a glimpse of the fiery chariot that enables us to travel through time and space, experiencing both the tranquillity of stillness and the vivacious flow of light and life. It's a magical moment that fills us with wonder and excitement, reminding us of the beauty and mystery of the universe.

The summer solstice occurs when the earth's tilt toward the sun is at a maximum and its highest position in the sky. On the day of the summer solstice, the Sun travels the longest path through the sky, and that day has the longest hours of daylight. Yellow is associated with the sun and its life-giving warmth and was one of the first colours used in art due to the wide availability of yellow ochre pigment.

According to Peter Carroll's *Liber Kaos*, "Yellow power has four distinct but related forms of manifestation within the psyche."

"The four aspects can be characterised as follows. Firstly the Ego, or self-image, is simply the model the mind has of the general personality, but excluding most of the extreme behaviour patterns that the selves are capable of. Secondly, Charisma is the degree of self-confidence that a person projects to others. Thirdly, something for which there is no single English term, but which can be called Laughter-Creativity. Fourthly, the urge to Assertion and Dominance. All these things are manifestations of the same yellow power; although their relative emphasis varies greatly between individuals." (Carroll: Liber Kaos)

The more I think about it, it seems to me that the colour Yellow is very much the Magician's colour. To walk the magician's path, one needs first to have charisma and then to integrate the Self with one's alter-ego and learn to use and project it when needed. A controlled alter-ego will result in powerful charisma and a strong sense of assertiveness and dominance in situations. We have all experienced the almost magical feeling when a charismatic person is walking into a room full of people. "The charismatic person is so confident and in control that it becomes impossible to refuse them anything." (Michael Kelly, The Satanic Dragon). Conversations will automatically cease in their presence, regardless of the importance, and people will eagerly provide assistance, direction or services without even being asked to.

Lyrical, Laughter & Creativity

For me, laughter and creativity correspond directly with the Lyrical, the 4th of the 5 rhythms dance system, created by Gabrielle Roth. Lyrical brings a jolt of motivation and elation, lifting us from the depths of disorder to a place of vigour and strength, rejuvenated and energized, stable and enabled.

The lyrical state speaks of creation, inspiration, rebirth and manifestation, like the shining hues of yellow emanating from the magician's aura. The colour yellow is linked to intellect and encourages us to tap into our creative potential. It guides our minds in finding solutions and making swift decisions, particularly when things become tense. It also promotes energy, optimism, self-belief, joviality, joyfulness, expectation and exhilaration. In addition, it stimulates neural pathways and glands, making us more perceptive and energised. Yellow improves memory recall and encourages communication through activity and interpersonal relationships.

Reading the above paragraph, it is hard to ignore the similarities and shared characteristics between the colour yellow and the Grapefruit essential oil.

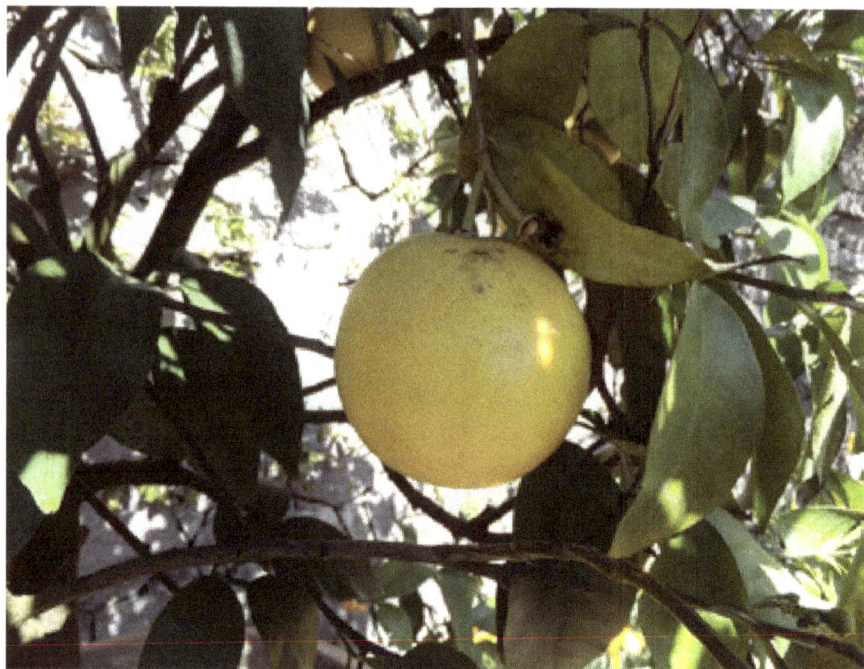

Grapefruit, Citrus x paradisi

(Photo courtesy of wiki commons wikimedia.org)

The Grapefruit is a cultivated tree, which often grows over 10 metres high and has glossy leaves and large yellow fruits. It is native to tropical Asia, and the West Indies; cultivated in California, Florida, Brazil and Israel. The oil is mainly produced in California.

Grapefruit has the power to energize and lift our mood, while simultaneously keeping us alert and focused. Its delicate yet distinct aroma offers a pleasant mix of sweetness with a slight hint of bitterness that helps us avoid becoming over-excited and displaying exaggerated emotional responses. I strongly recommend using Grapefruit essential oil to help you focus on studying, writing, or driving. Just put two drops on a tissue and smell it when needed. For further reading about the Grapefruit, look up *2023: A Trilogy by The Justified Ancient of Mu Mu.*

The Sun and Gold both possess a yellow hue and are thought to be everlasting, unchanging and unbreakable. It was believed that the gods were created from gold, so figurines in their honour were crafted of or simply gilded with this precious metal. Furthermore, masks covering mummies and royal sarcophagi were usually made with gold. Ra, an ancient Egyptian deity, is a prominent figure in the pantheon. He is the ruler of all gods and the creator of all beings, as well as a guardian of power, kingship, sun and illumination. Not only does he control the activity of the sun, but Ra can even be considered the tangible embodiment of it.

Akhenaten was an Egyptian pharaoh who ruled during the Eighteenth Dynasty of the New Kingdom period of Ancient Egypt. He is the earliest known creator of a new religion. The cult he founded broke from the

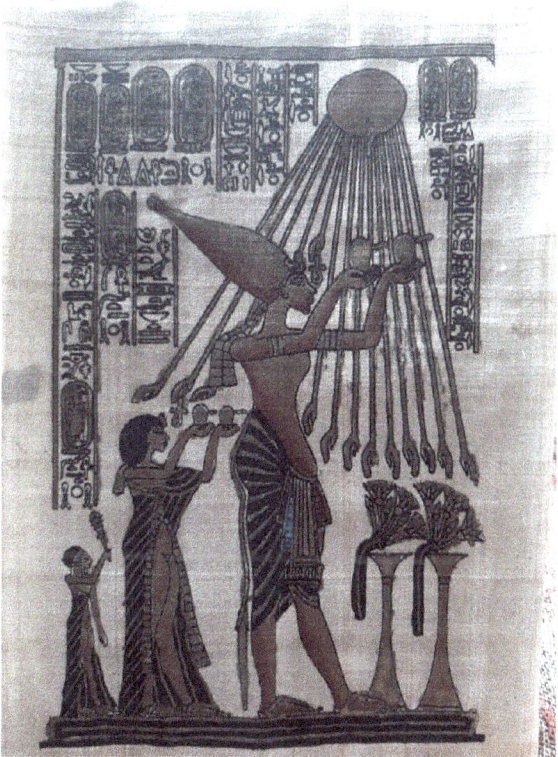

traditional polytheism of ancient Egypt and focused on the worship of a single god named Aten. Aten, a Sun god, is depicted as the solar disk emitting rays terminating in human hands, which was an aspect of Ra. Akhenaten identified himself with the sun god Aten and elevated the cult of Aten above the worship of most other gods, including Amon, the king of the gods.

Beautiful, you appear
in the horizon of the sky,
oh, living sun,
who determines life!
You have appeared on the eastern horizon
and filled every land with your beauty.
You are beautiful, great and shining,
high over all the land.
Your rays embrace the lands
to the limit of all you have created.
You are Ra when you reach their borders
and bow them down to your beloved son.
You are distant, though your rays are on earth;
you are in their face, though your course is inscrutable …
From "The Great Hymn to the Aten"

Akhenaten saw himself as Aten's earthly manifestation, and as such, in his mind and his followers' eyes, he was the Sun, the protector and healer, the epitome of success, physical energy and magical power. These characteristics bring to mind Helichrysum, another plant which is ruled by the sun, a plant whose healing properties have been touched by the everlasting essence of the immortality of the Sun's gold. I've already discussed the qualities and benefits of this fantastic plant in an earlier chapter, so I will not repeat myself. However, for those of you who want to go deeper and learn more about "The lost history of Immortelle, the Everlasting Flower" I highly recommend Elizabeth Ashley's book: *Helichrysum For The Wound That Will Not Heal.*

Every time I hear someone using this phrase, "There is nothing new under the Sun" (Ecclesiastes 1:9) I can't help but ponder the hidden message of this sentence. To make sense of things, we have to start with the creation of the sun.

The creation myth in both the Pyramid Texts and the Bible starts with very similar ideas. In the beginning, there was the primaeval waters of chaos and then, according to the Bible, God created the sun. According to the Pyramid Texts, the world was said to have emerged from an infinite, lifeless sea when the sun rose for the first time. Ra/Atum (both being creator/sun gods), emerged from a chaotic state of the world and gave rise to Shu (air) and Tefnut (moisture), from their union came Geb (earth) and Nut (sky), who in turn created Osiris, Isis, Set, Nephthys and Horus the elder.

By the Fifth Dynasty, in the 25th and 24th centuries bce, Ra had become one of the most important gods in ancient Egyptian religion, identified primarily with the noon-day sun. Ra ruled in all parts of the created world: the sky, the earth, and the underworld. Because of the life-giving qualities of the sun, the Egyptians worshipped the sun as a god. The creator of the universe and the giver of life, the sun or Ra represented life, warmth and growth. As the sun god, one of his duties was to carry the sun across the sky on his solar barque to light the day. But when twilight came he and his vessel travelled to the underworld, he would have to sail and cross through the twelve gates and regions. Every night Apophis attacked Ra and attempted to stop the Sun boat's progress.

When Ra travelled in his Sun boat, he was accompanied by Set, who overcame the serpent Apep.

Apep, also called Apophis, was the personification of chaos and Ra's arch-enemy. He was said to lie just below the horizon line, trying to devour the sun as Ra travelled through the underworld. After Set defeats Apophis, Ra would leave the underworld, returning, and again illuminating the day. The role of the god Set in Egyptian mythology is to make sure that at the end of each night, the sun will again rise and become. In my humble opinion, this is the essence of the phrase: There is nothing new under the Sun.

No matter what we do, think, invent or build, at the end of the day, it's the same old 'life versus death' survival race, darkness falls and chaos lurks at the corners and wants to swallow the sun. But at the end of every night, for as long as Set, the Dark Lord of Chaos keeps slaying the primaeval serpent Apophis, The Sun, with all his might and glory, will rise and shine on a new day.

In the mornings
when I wake up
by your side
two suns rise in my eyes
Shining light so bright
I can see your body
sparkle with golden dust,
I could see your heart
melting into the stones
When we kissed under the
Golden Dawn

Summer Solstice ritual

According to the Tantric and Egyptian-Tantra tradition, there are four twilights: Dawn-east, Noon-south, Dusk-west, and Midnight-north.

In Liber Resh, Aleister Crowley wrote the four adorations to the Sun which should perform according to the four twilights mentioned above.

Liber Resh was written for the Syllabus of the official AA and its purpose was to prepare the mind for meditation, to help to manage our practices, to learn how to centre ourselves, to draw force from the sun and conquer death, and how to connect with nature. Liber Resh aims for the daily practice of the four adorations.

Liber Resh vel Helios
sub figura CC
Publication in class D

0.   These are the adorations to be performed by aspirants to the Argentium Astrum (order of the Silver Star)

1   Let him greet the Sun at dawn, facing East, giving the sign of his grade. And let him say in a loud voice:
    Hail unto Thee who art Ra in Thy rising, even unto Thee who art Ra in Thy strength, who travellest over the Heavens in Thy bark at the Uprising of the Sun.
    Tahuti standeth in His splendour at the prow, and Ra-Hoor abideth at the helm.
    Hail unto Thee from the Abodes of Night!

2.   Also at Noon, let him greet the Sun, facing South, giving the sign of his grade. And let him say in a loud voice:

Hail unto Thee who art Ahathoor in Thy triumphing, even unto Thee who art Ahathoor in Thy beauty, who travellest over the heavens in thy bark at the Mid-course of the Sun.

Tahuti standeth in His splendour at the prow, and Ra-Hoor abideth at the helm.

Hail unto Thee from the Abodes of Morning!

3.   Also, at Sunset, let him greet the Sun, facing West, giving the sign of his grade. And let him say in a loud voice:

Hail unto Thee who art Tum in Thy setting, even unto Thee who art Tum in Thy joy, who travellest over the Heavens in Thy bark at the Down-going of the Sun.

Tahuti standeth in His splendour at the prow, and Ra-Hoor abideth at the helm.

Hail unto Thee from the Abodes of Day!

4.   Lastly, at Midnight, let him greet the Sun, facing North, giving the sign of his grade, and let him say in a loud voice:

Hail unto thee who art Khephra in Thy hiding, even unto Thee who art Khephra in Thy silence, who travellest over the heavens in Thy bark at the Midnight Hour of the Sun.

Tahuti standeth in His splendour at the prow, and Ra-Hoor abideth at the helm.

Hail unto Thee from the Abodes of Evening.

5.   And after each of these invocations thou shalt give the sign of silence, and afterward thou shalt perform the adoration that is taught thee by thy Superior. And then do thou compose Thyself to holy meditation.

6. Also it is better if in these adorations thou assume the God-form of Whom thou adorest, as if thou didst unite with Him in the adoration of That which is beyond Him.

7. Thus shalt thou ever be mindful of the Great Work which thou hast undertaken to perform, and thus shalt thou be strengthened to pursue it unto the attainment of the Stone of the Wise, the Summum Bonum, True Wisdom and Perfect Happiness.

* * *

The Morgan Witches' tradition of Sun adoration started a few years ago on a summer solstice Dusk to Dawn ritual at Stonehenge. Each year since then, we celebrate a different twilight. This year we celebrated the Sun in the West at sunset. Usually, we would greet the Sun on higher ground, a hill or a mountain. This year, we decided that the perfect location would be somewhere by the sea to salute the Sun in its glorious setting in the west.

Once we found our perfect spot for the ritual, we placed our Ra avatars all around us. Ra avatars can be anything that symbolises the sun, it could be traditional or universal symbols of the sun or a personalised one. In The Litany of Ra, a clay figurine of Ra is used for the ritual. My suggestion is to take a bottle of Helichrysum/Grapefruit essential oil and smell it between the verses. If you are by the sea, you can also collect some pebbles and shells and draw or paint Sun symbols on them.

We open the ritual with the sunset adoration from Liber Resh:

3. Also, at Sunset, let him greet the Sun, facing West, giving the sign of his grade. And let him say in a loud voice:

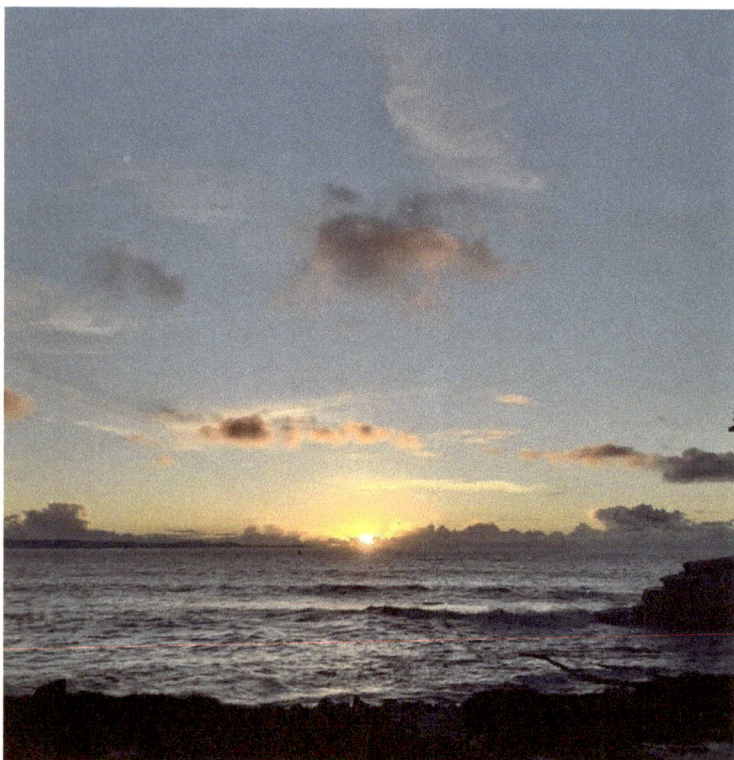

Hail unto Thee who art Tum in Thy setting, even unto Thee who art Tum in Thy joy, who travellest over the Heavens in Thy bark at the Down-going of the Sun. Tahuti standeth in His splendour at the prow, and Ra-Hoor abideth at the helm. Hail unto Thee from the Abodes of Day!

We inhale the essences of the Sun and salute it, and then carry on reading The Litany of Ra while stopping to inhale from the essences of the sun between each of the verses.

The Litany of RA

(Canto 1, edited from *Egyptian Magick*, Mogg Morgan:2021)

Title: The beginning of the book of the worship of RA in the West, (The heavenly region) of the worship of the United One in the West.

When anyone reads this book, clay figures of the avatar of Ra are placed upon the ground, at the hour of the setting of the Sun, that is of the triumph of RA over his enemies in the West.

1. Homage to thee, RA ! Supreme power, the master of the hidden spheres who causes the principles to arise, who dwells in darkness, who is born as the all surrounding universe.

2. Homage to thee, RA ! Supreme power, the beetle that folds his wings, that rests in the empyrean, that is born as his son.

3. Homage to thee, RA ! Supreme power, TANEN (The Earth) who produces his members (Gods), who fashions what is in him, who is born within his sphere.

4. Homage to thee, RA ! Supreme power, he who discloses the earth and lights the Ament, he whose principle has (become) his manifestation, and who is born under the form of the god with the large disk.

5. Homage to thee, RA ! Supreme power, the soul that speaks, that rests upon her high place, that creates the hidden intellects which are developed in her.

6. Homage to thee, RA ! Supreme power, the only one, the courageous one, who fashions his body, he who calls his gods (to life), when he arrives in his hidden sphere.

7. Homage to thee, RA ! Supreme power, he who addresses his eye, and who speaks to himself, he who imparts the breath of life to the souls (that are) in their place; they receive it and develop.

8. Homage to thee, RA ! Supreme power, the spirit that walks, that destroys its enemies, that sends pain to the rebels.

9. Homage to thee, RA ! Supreme power, he who shines when he is in his sphere, who sends his darkness into his sphere, and who hides what it contains.

10. Homage to thee, RA ! Supreme power, he who lights the bodies which are on the horizon, he who enters his sphere.

Salute the sun and say your thanks.

16. Red Magick
Lammas

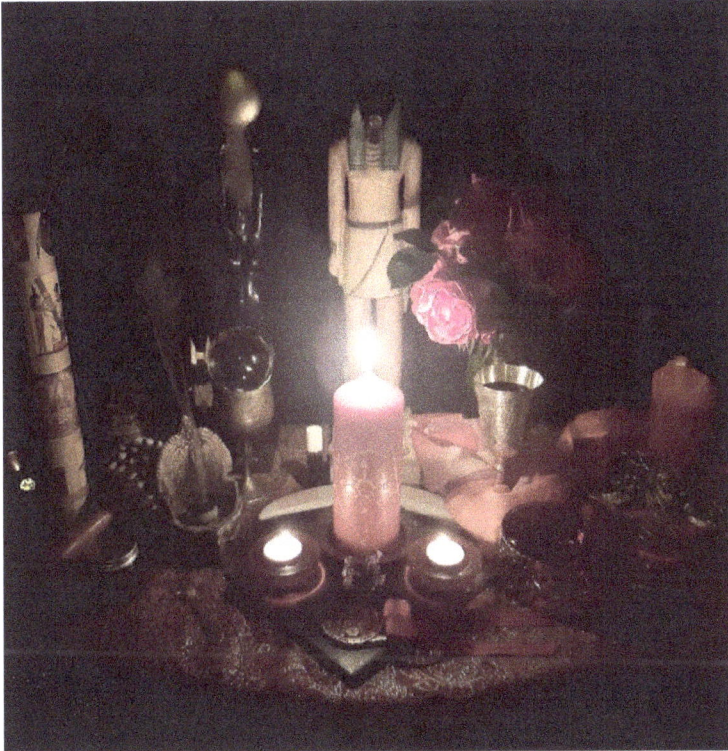

At Lammas, we arrive at the peak of the summer months. Like the other quarterly festivals, Samhain, Imbolc & Beltane, Lammas represents the change in energy. The cool and clear energy of Yellow Magick has turned into a hot, sweltering, wild red energy. Lammas is the year's gate in which we can connect to the red energy. It is the time to cut, break and reap all the destructive elements in our lives and harvest our 'summer crops' and 'burn' the stuff we no longer need.

The colour red is a symbolic representation of many different emotions and feelings. It stands for blood, fire, love, passion, warmth, romance, joy, power, courage, willpower, rage, anger, danger and stress. Red is also associated with sensuality and leadership.

> "Red magic has two aspects, firstly the invocation of the vitality, aggression, and morale to sustain oneself in any conflict from life in general to outright war, and secondly the conduct of actual combat magic ... However, the real skill of red magic is to be able to present such an overwhelming glamour of personal vitality, morale and potential for aggression that the exercise of combat magic is never required." (Carroll 1992)

With this in mind, I always felt that the red magick season is the best time of the year to connect with our inner demons and face our fears, frustrations, obsessions, jealousy, self-criticism and resentment. One should try to find a way to integrate and channel all those raw and explosive energies for your own benefit.

Red magick meets us at the height of the summer when the Dog Days are upon us. The term "Dog Days" traditionally refers to a period of particularly hot and humid weather occurring during the summer months of July and August in the Northern Hemisphere. Historically, the period following the heliacal rising of Sirius (the "Dog Star") was known for its connection to heat, drought, sudden thunderstorms, lethargy, fever, mad dogs and according to Hellenistic astrology, bad luck. Today, this part of summer is said to be the most sweltering and uncomfortable in the Northern Hemisphere. Those sizzling summer days resonate with the fire element and its spicy scents.

Action, vibration, glow, determination and assertiveness. Sex, breaking habits, purification, protection, aggression and strength, are the keywords that correspond with the energy of red magick and its fiery nature. Red magick can be employed to fan the flames of the kundalini power, the wellspring of our creativity and ingenious ideas. If we concentrate on intense emotions like malice and envy, or on hexes, they will simply splinter back at us and keep us stuck in a loop.

But by channelling the fiery energy of red magick towards gaining vigour and inventiveness, we are able to open up paths out of complex predicaments and progress. It is likely too hot for a bath ritual in such weather so I contemplated the best way to tie into the fiery and dry energies of the season would be by crafting a spell jar to hold and direct all the 'demons' I mentioned earlier, to be used when we need an extra push of strength and confidence. We will be working with dry herbs and spices representing the energy of fire, gathering their magickal qualities into a potion specifically to wield red magick. This potion may be used whenever we require a surge of red magick.

Red Magick potion

To make your potion, you will need a small or medium size bottle (I recommend not less than 30 ml and no more than ½ a litre).

Dried or powdered ginger

Cinnamon stick

Black pepper (I recommend using the dry peppercorn but if no other option, black pepper powder will do too).

Dry Basil leaves

Clove

Dried orange peel

A bottle of red food colouring.

Enough Vodka/White Rum to fill up the potion bottle.

Red tablecloth

Knife

Mortar

A little cutting board

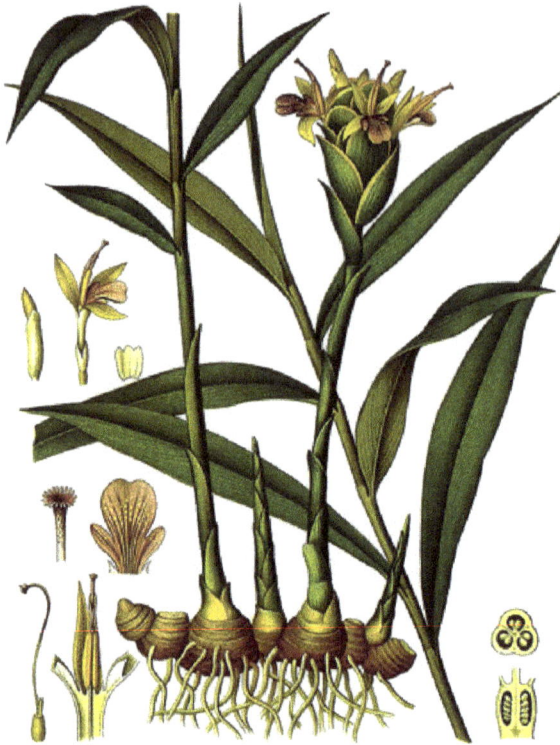

Ginger, Zingiber officinale

(Photo courtesy of wiki commons wikimedia.org)

A tropical perennial herb that can grow up to 1 metre high with a very pungent and thick, tuberous rhizome root from which both the essential oil and the spice are extracted. Ginger is native to Southeast Asia.

The sweet woody, warm-spicy scent has a stimulating effect on our body and mind. One of Ginger's main therapeutic qualities is as a digestive stimulant helping to restore our physical and spiritual appetite. Its hot and fiery characteristics are the force and drive behind our magical and physical energy and give us the courage to get up and create a better life filled with love and security for ourselves.

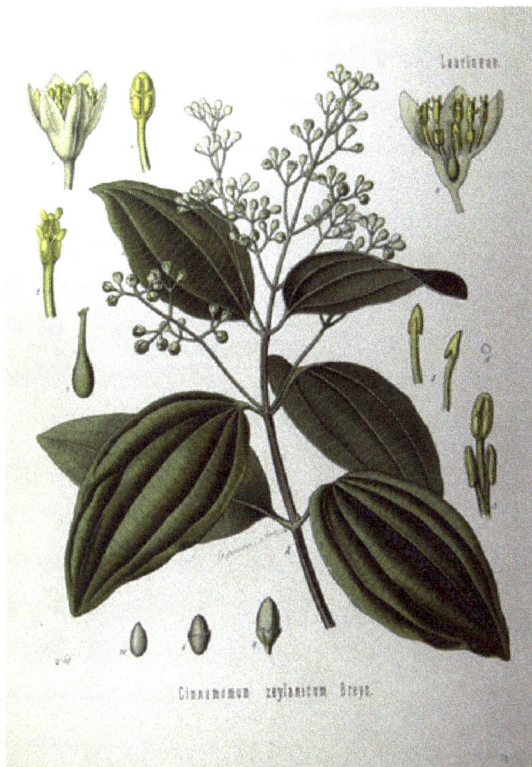

Cinnamon, Cinnamomum zeylanicum

(Photo courtesy of wiki commons wikimedia.org)

A tropical tree up to 15 metres high, with strong branches and thick scabrous bark. Cinnamon is native to Sri Lanka, Madagascar, the Comoro Islands, South India, Myanmar and Indochina.

Like Ginger, Cinnamon has a warm, sweet and spicy aroma that strengthens and energies our physical, mental and psychic awareness and well-being.

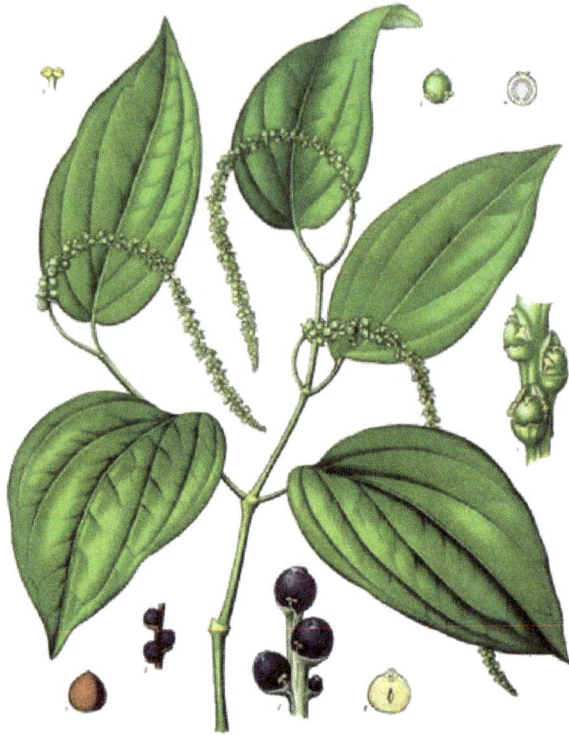

Black Pepper, Piper nigrum

(Photo courtesy of wiki commons wikimedia.org)

Black pepper is a flowering vine in the Piperaceae family. The fruit is a drupe which is about 5 mm in diameter, dark red and contains a stone which encloses a single pepper seed. Black pepper is native to the Malabar Coast of India.

The powerful and sharp aroma of Black pepper promotes mental alertness and initiates protection, it also stimulates and energises and gives us the courage and strength to deal with precarious risky situations.

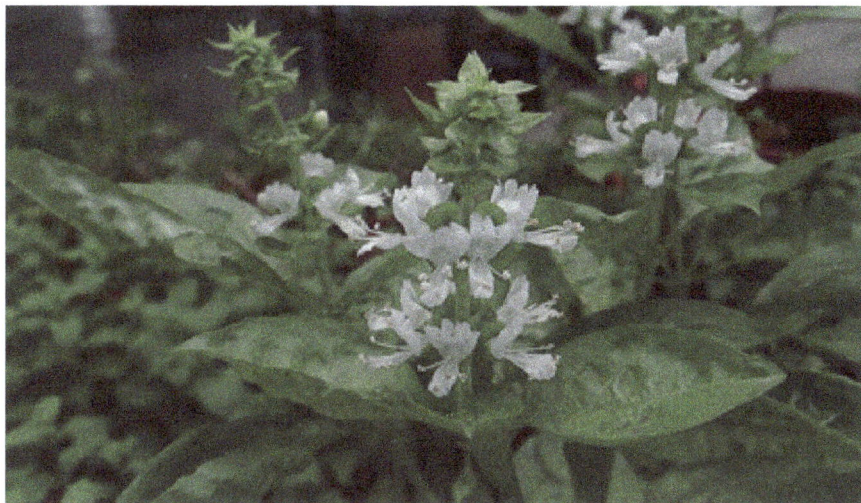

Basil, Ocimum basilicum

(Photo courtesy of wiki commons wikimedia.org)

A tender annual herb, with dark green leaves, and greyish-green beneath, can rise to 60 cm with small white flowers. Basil is native to tropical Asia and Africa, it is now widely cultivated throughout Europe, the Mediterranean, the Pacific Islands, North and South America.

The strong spicy fragrance uplifts the spirits and clears the mind helping us in the process of decision-making. The rich scent and the lushness of its green colour suggestive of Basil's long association with money spells and wealth magick.

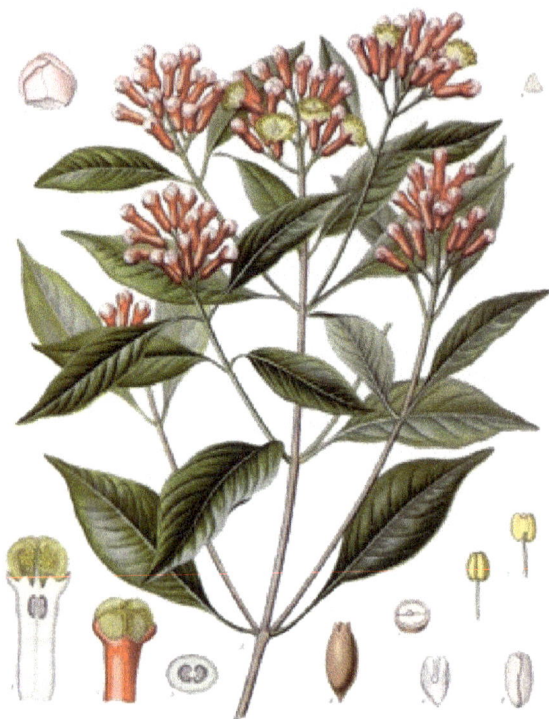

Clove, Syzygium aromaticum

(Photo courtesy of wiki commons wikimedia.org)

A slender evergreen tree with a smooth grey trunk that can grow up to 12 metres with large bright green leaves. Clove is native to Indonesia and is now cultivated worldwide.

A sweet-spicy and fruity aroma that vibrates on the scale of the top notes. Clove's unusual scent (very spicy but noticeably light at the same time) seems to penetrate the darkest corners of our minds, helping us to retrieve and remember forgotten information and lost details. Its healing and analgesic properties are well known and have been used around the world for toothache, skin infections and much more for over 2000 years.

The clove-penetrating aroma can be assigned as an energetic protective agent. In our Red Magick blend, clove plays the part of both the healer and the protector.

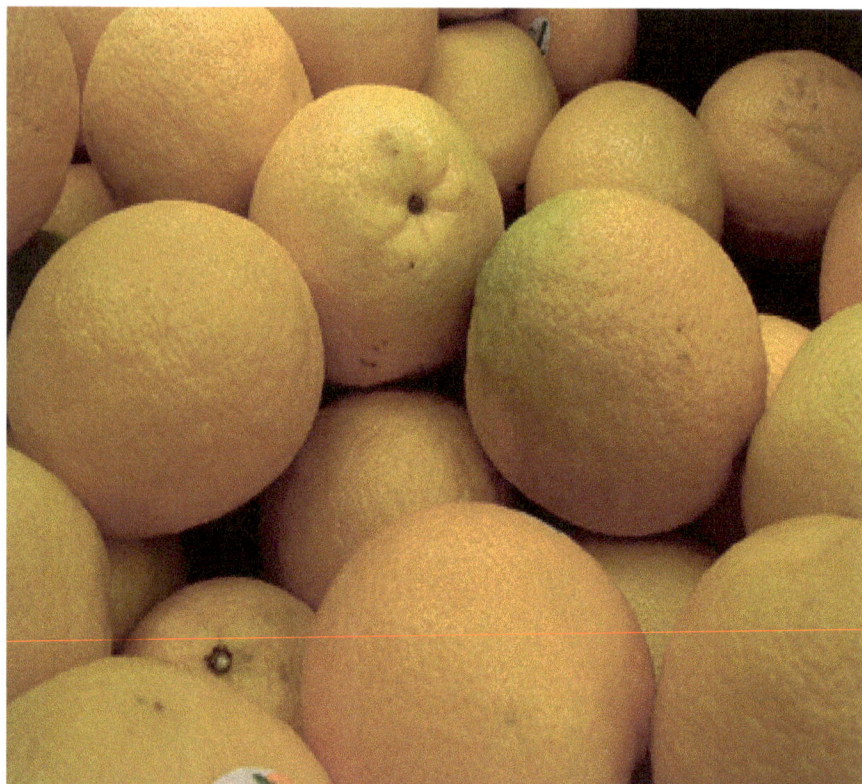

Orange, Citrus sinensis

(Photo courtesy of wiki commons wikimedia.org)

A small evergreen tree with sweet fruit and non-bitter membranes. The Orange is native to China; extensively cultivated especially in the USA (California and Florida) and around the Mediterranean.

The sweet and citrusy fragrance of the Orange has an immediate effect, transforming our mood and lifting our spirits. It opens our hearts and filling them with joy and cleansing our aura

* * *

It is important to set aside some uninterrupted time for yourself before beginning the process of making your potion. This way, you can fully concentrate and approach the task with a clear and focused mind. When you are ready to prepare your potion, close the door behind you and start tuning to the frequencies and energies of the ingredients, the herbs, alcohol, and food colouring that you are going to put into the bottle. Arrange all your ingredients on the red tablecloth and start to prepare the spices.

Cut a piece of the ginger and the orange into small chunks, put the peppercorn into the mortar, crush them and set them aside, do the same with the cloves and cinnamon, smell the Basil and crush a bit of it between your fingers. While you are doing so, take a couple of moments to get acquainted with each spice, feel its texture, and smell the aroma.

Once you have done it, it is time to prepare mentally for the task ahead. Sit and meditate for a few minutes, and try to find your core, your strength. Remember, you are dealing with very spicy and hot plants, sentient beings. You need to be extremely focused and clear as a crystal with your intentions when you put each one of them into your bottle. I always think of my potions as Genies in bottles. To 'master' them you need to learn as much as you can about their uses and characteristics, to get them to 'work for you and do your will, you need to respect them and treat them with honour.

When you are ready, take a deep breath and say the following spell (Morgan 2021) loud and clear.

I invoke and beseech the consecration,
O gods of the heavens
O gods under the earth
O gods circling on the middle region from one womb

O masters of all the living and dead

O heedful in many necessities of gods and men

O concealers of things now seen

O directors of Isis, Nemesis and Adrasteia

who spend every hour with you

O senders of fate who travels around the whole world

O commanders of the rulers

O exalters of the abased

O revealers of the hidden

O guides of the winds

O arousers of the waves

O bringers of fire at the appropriate time

O creators and benefactors of every race

O Lords and controllers of kings

Come, benevolent ones, for the purpose for which I call you,

as benevolent assistants in this rite for my benefit.

Who moulded the forms of the beasts of the Zodiac

Who found their routes

Who was the begetter of fruits?

Who raises up the mountains?

Who made the winds hold to their annual tasks

What Aion nourishing an Aion rules the Aions?

One deathless god

You are the begetter of all and assign souls to all

and control all,

King of the Aions and Lord before who

mountains and plains

springs and rivers

valleys of earth

spirits and all things

High shining heaven

and every sea trembles.

Lord, ruler of all, the holy one

and master of all.

By your power, the elements exist

and all things come into being,

the route of the sun and moon,

of night and dawn

all things in air and earth and water and fire.

Yours is the eternal processional way of [heaven]

in which the seven-lettered name is established for the harmony of the seven sounds of the planets which utter their voices according to the phases of the moon.

You give wealth, good old age, good children, strength, and food.

You lord of life, ruler of the upper and lower realm,

whose justice is not thwarted,

whose glorious name the angels' hymn,

who have the truth that never lies,

hear me and complete for me this operation so that I may wear this power in every place,

in every time, without being smitten or afflicted,

so as to be preserved intact from every danger

while I wear this power.

Yea lord, for to you,

the god in heaven,

all things are subject, and none of the daimons or spirits will oppose me

because I have called on your great name for the consecration.

The gates of heaven are opened

The gates of the earth are opened

The route of the sea is opened

The route of the rivers is opened

My spirit is heard by gods and daemons

My spirit is heard by the spirit of heaven

My spirit is heard by the terrestrial spirit

My spirit is heard by the marine spirit

My spirit is heard by the riverine spirit

Therefore give spirit to the Red Magick Potion

I have prepared

O gods whom I have named and called on

Give breath to the Red Magick Potion

Let its mouth be opened

so that it may breathe and live

According to the Egyptian way: Ei IEOU - Oh Hail

According to the Jews: Ei IEOU - Oh Hail

According to the Greeks: Ei IEOU - Oh Hail

According to the High Priests of Egypt: Ei IEOU - Oh Hail

According to the Hindus - Ei IEOU - Oh Hail

Consecrate and empower this Red Magick Potion for me,

for the entire and glorious time of my life.

I suggest customising the following words to suit you. Whatever fits your style and preferences is what you should use. Making them yours will allow for a more effective outcome.

Put your Ginger in the bottle and say:

The potent root, Ginger, fortifies both my physical and spiritual being, aiding me in acquiring the ability to both give and receive love, for both myself and those around me.

Add Cinnamon to the bottle and say:

May the sweet and spicy scent of cinnamon enhance my physical vitality and expand my mental clarity, ushering abundance and prosperity into my life while teaching me how to maintain it.

Add Black Pepper to the bottle and say:
Black Pepper, a mighty warrior and protector, defender of the realm and space beyond, give me the strength and courage to stand in the face of danger and overcome my fears and obstacles on my path.

Add Basil and say:
Holy Basil, I humbly seek your guidance and insight. Please impart your ancient wisdom upon me and help me gain clarity of mind and vision. Remove any limiting beliefs that hinder me from reaching my full potential.

Add Clove and say:
Clove, ancient healer, I ask for your help to bring light into the darkest corners of my mind. Please help me retrieve and sharpen lost memories, restore my health and heal my pain.

When all five Genies have been placed inside the bottle, fill it to the brim and add a few drops of the red food colouring until a satisfactory hue is achieved. Ensure that everything is well mixed by stirring and shaking well, then seal the bottle neatly and put it on your altar. This will permit it to be further charged with the currents of Red Magick energy.

Disclaimer

The Red Magick potion is a powerful spell; you resort to it only after you have exhausted all other options in the face of a difficult situation. The more you use it, however, the less effective it will be, as its potency will decrease. Think of the five Genies in the bottle - that's how strong this spell can be!

I cannot give you definitive instructions on what occasions, the quantity or the implications of using this potion. However, I am confident that when the moment arrives, you will know what to do. You should also consider that if you don't evaluate the situation properly, the potion might have an adverse effect.

Lastly, if you choose to go ahead and create the concoction, remember that it was made by you and for you only. It is impossible to ascertain the impact it might have on anyone else who consumes it.

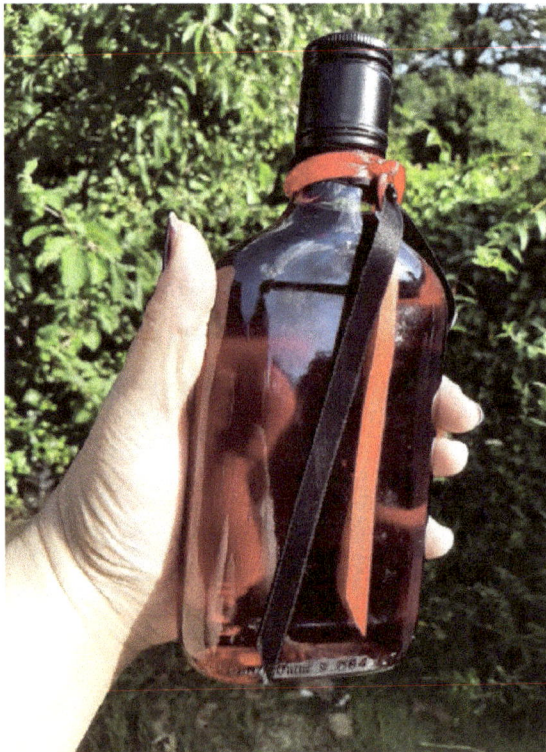

17. Blue Magick
Autumn Equinox

This chapter is dedicated to all the Jewitches out there. May our voices be heard and balance out all the haters, extremists and deniers of the truth.

To Sophia,

From Thunder Perfect Mind

Translated by George W. MacRae.

I was sent forth from the power,

and I have come to those who reflect upon me,

and I have been found among those who seek after me.

Look upon me, you who reflect upon me,

and you hearers, hear me.

You who are waiting for me, take me to yourselves.

And do not banish me from your sight.

And do not make your voice hate me, nor your hearing.

Do not be ignorant of me anywhere or any time. Be on your guard!

Do not be ignorant of me.

For I am the first and the last.

I am the honoured one and the scorned one.

I am the whore and the holy one.

I am the wife and the virgin.

I am the mother and the daughter.

I am the members of my mother.

I am the barren one

and many are her sons.

I am she whose wedding is great,

and I have not taken a husband.

I am the midwife and she who does not bear.

I am the solace of my labour pains.

I am the bride and the bridegroom,

and it is my husband who begot me.

I am the mother of my father

and the sister of my husband

and he is my offspring.

I am the slave of him who prepared me.

I am the ruler of my offspring.

But he is the one who begot me before the time on a birthday.

And he is my offspring in (due) time,

and my power is from him.

I am the staff of his power in his youth,

and he is the rod of my old age.

And whatever he wills happens to me.

I am the silence that is incomprehensible

and the idea whose remembrance is frequent.

I am the voice whose sound is manifold

and the word whose appearance is multiple.

I am the utterance of my name.

Why, you who hate me, do you love me,

and hate those who love me?

You who deny me, confess me,

and you who confess me, deny me.

You who tell the truth about me, lie about me,

and you who have lied about me, tell the truth about me.

You who know me, be ignorant of me,

and those who have not known me, let them know me.

For I am knowledge and ignorance.

I am shame and boldness.

I am shameless; I am ashamed.

I am strength and I am fear.

I am war and peace.

Give heed to me.

The wheel of the year never stops or rests. The glorious warmth of summer is now a distant memory, and evening temperatures have dropped. It's hard to believe that only yesterday we were celebrating red magick. Autumn is a time to give thanks for the abundance of the land. We can marvel at the ripening of fruit and the vastness of our harvest. It's an occasion to rejoice in all that Mother Nature has provided. Yet, it's also a reminder that this season symbolises decay, decline, ageing, and death - if we don't collect and store our crops now, we won't benefit from their yield later.

Twice a year the wheel stops for a moment when the sun is situated exactly above the equator and day and night are of equal length. This happens on the Spring and Autumn Equinoxes. During the autumnal equinox, the sun shines directly on the equator, and the northern and southern hemispheres get the same amount of rays. This is the perfect time to find again the balance between our physical and spiritual lives, letting go of all we don't need anymore and creating a more sustainable space in our hearts and homes for the abundance of the last of the harvest.

On this autumn equinox, we were blessed to welcome a new addition to our coven, so on behalf of baby Sophia and her mom, we started our ritual with an invocation for a safe passage and arrival of mother and child.

Tawaret/Ipet is the Egyptian goddess protector of the household, childbirth and children in general as her name suggests - Ipet = The Nurse.

Ipet Invocation

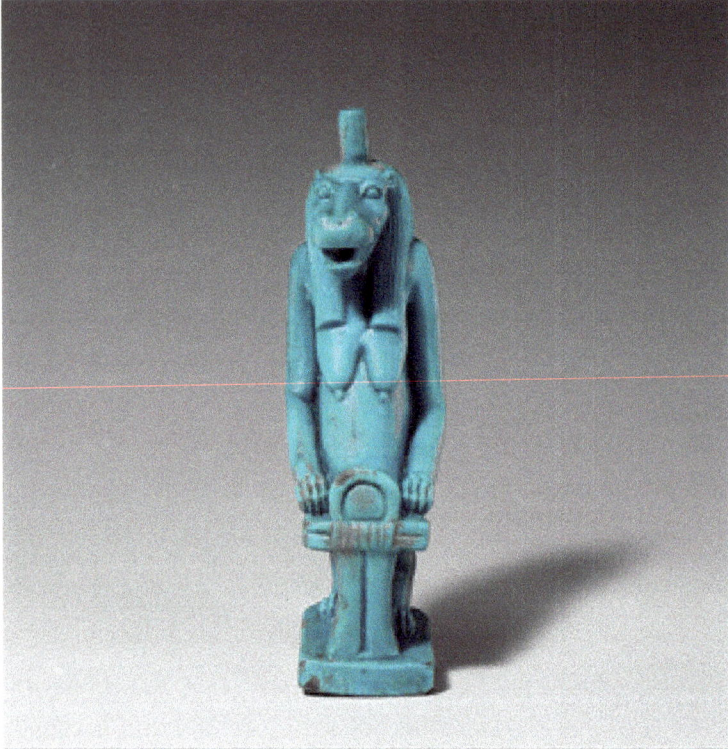

(Photo courtesy of wiki commons wikimedia.org)

Awake and embrace the void

Your heart is strong enough for its joys

and its worries Leave,

and when you awake to life

You will feel young again on the new day Rest,

lie down assured of long good health.

"Good night,

the gods protect you,

their protection is before you each day

No bad thing approaches

The demon (Apep) is repelled from your bed chamber

Ipet the Great protects you in your long and powerful life."

The day and night illumined,

You shine forth

For she guides your steps on the right path,

And you know what is needed,

The god Ptah provisions you,

filling your storeroom,

With food and drink aplenty,

and in good measure.

Your diary and records are all in order

and well-composed.

The mistakes of the past are forgotten,

and the staff in your hand is well-made and sustaining.

Break bread with the wise,

Your cares all behind you.

Only reason lies before you,

The best is yet to come.

*

Praise be to TAWERET,

Bringing 'perfection' in her beautiful name.

I praise her to the limits of the sky,

I desire her Ka, calming day by day.

Be merciful to me,

May I behold your mercy,

You, of perfect mercy!

Extend your hand to me,

Giving me life,

And granting me offspring!

Do not reproach me for my errors

You, in perfect mercy!

Even if my helpers slip up,

My peers still reward me.

I desire your great strength,

None knows you as I do;

I will say to the children and children's children:

Thee as guardian before her!

Joy my heart should seize,

Because on this day TAWERET is merciful,

My house prospers with her blessings.

May she give them day after day,

And I never say 'Oh I have regrets!'

May she continue to give me health,

And my womb bears children safely,

[Or the future be secure].

My heart is glad every day, for sure

The good ones expel the evil,

And I am blessed.

Behold her people will live forever,

My enemies are fearful before you TAWARET!

Since your rage oppresses them

more than a mountain of iron,

Her mercy gives us life!

> I am the blue-lidded daughter of Sunset; I am the naked
> brilliance of the voluptuous night-sky.

> Liber AL 1:64

Blue is a colour that symbolizes the sky above us and the sea beneath us.

It is a representation of the expanse around us, from the heavens to the depths of the ocean.

Blue is a colour that speaks to liberation, imagination, intuitive perception, creativity, depth and tenderness. It also invites thoughts of trustworthiness, truthfulness, intelligence, faithfulness, steadiness and equilibrium. These qualities are reflective of blue magic - the season of bounty and equilibrium.

Blue magick coincides with the Jewish holiday period, representing prosperity and equilibrium. On Rosh Hashanah, we observe the start of a new cycle, being thankful for what has been and wishing for a prosperous forthcoming year. Yom Kippur then follows, the most sacred Jewish day, focusing on repentance and prayer; hoping that our hearts will be as light as a feather and justice will side with us so our names may be written in the book of life. Just a few days after Yom Kippur, the autumnal celebration continues with the eight-day festival of Sukkot. This holiday offers a combination of significance and the chance to form meaningful connections. It is the ideal occasion to achieve harmony and balance.

Sukkot is a time for celebrating the harmony between our core beliefs as a group. We rejoice in the abundance of the land and how much it contributes to our lives, whilst being aware of how temporary and fragile life can be. This balance of joy and respect creates an atmosphere of appreciation for our faith and community.

> "You shall dwell in sukkot seven days ... in order that future generations may know that I made the Israelite people live in sukkot when I brought them out of the land of Egypt, I the Lord your God." (Leviticus 23:42)

Sukkot marks our connection to the story of the Israelites' exodus from Egypt. No matter how much time has passed, it seems that our bond with this ancient land never truly severed. We can observe the lasting impact Egypt had on us through many of our traditions and customs, particularly Yom Kippur; a day when we are judged by God and must atone for our actions. Here, I cannot help but draw parallels between what we practise today and what the Egyptians believed thousands of years ago, that upon death one shall appear before Goddess Ma'at where the heart is weighed against her white feather on a scale of justice.

Ma'at - the Essence of Balance

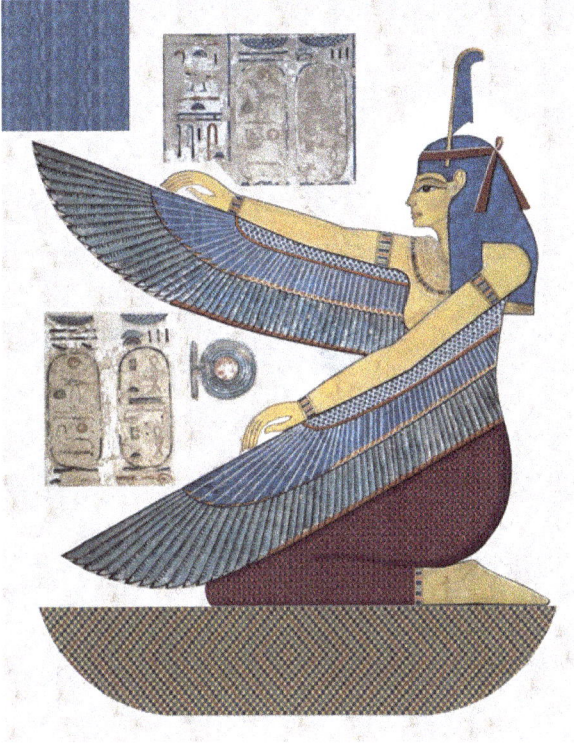

By Mogg Morgan (2023)

(Photo courtesy of wiki commons wikimedia.org)

The concept of Ma'at means "the reward of an agent lies in what is done for him. That's the ultimate god for Maat." (From an inscription of Neferhote.) Which looks very like the later concept of Karma. This would make it almost an inner law of the cosmos, like cause and effect, natural. Everything is connected in such a way that whatever action one takes, will have consequences. Being in a state of balance is self-evidently for the best, and one's actions in life should be those that do not radically disrupt this or cause it to disappear, or harmony will be replaced by entropy and system breakdown. The system is robust enough to cope with, and may even require some anarchy to keep it healthy and flexible, but too much and things fall apart disastrously.

Egypt had no strict law code as such. There are some lists of rules that can be viewed as a code, but this is far from certain if it ever really was a law code like the Ten Commandments or Laws of Hammurabi. It seems more likely that the right actions and values were self-evident. In our hearts, we know when we are being straight and when we are being crooked. In terms of etymology, the original meaning of Maat suggests straightness, straight but certainly not square.

Thus it says in one important magical text "As the representative of the divine law of order, truth and justice or Ma'at is the Ba is our true inner voice." (Kriekamp, Amduat, Introduction). It is about listening to our hearts. This I would say is also what the message of the Thelemic holy book Liber AL is also about. There is no sin, there is no guilt, and only one law, do what you wilt. This means following your refined inner sense of the straight path of the wise, and this is the only rule you and anyone else may ever need. It may seem idealistic, but for a long time, this system of natural law was all the Egyptians needed, it worked well for them.

The counterpart of Ma'at is Isfet or wrongdoing. This evolved to personal rather than communal value, more like the concept of Sin, an offence against the will of god. Community values became an arbitrary, personal revelation from god, what pleases them, which had to be interpreted by specialists. The more communal way seems better to me. Follow one's own heart, with love and understanding. Whatever one does, should not, on balance, damage the whole. This singular rule applies to all, gods and people. Even the magician, aiming for the "goal of the wise" will maintain

Ma'at. Another older name for Ma'at was lioness Tefnut, who was paired with the lionine god Shu.

Coffin Text spells 75-80, distinguished between cosmology and biogony, creator god and life god. Atum was the creator of the world and life according to this theology, but the task of life-giving and developing both fell to his two children Shu and Tefnut. In this capacity, Shu received the name Ankh "life" and was called "endless time", while Tefnut was called Ma'at "truth/justice/order" and Djet "invariable permanence".

There is a fourfold blessing of Shu's cosmic winds from the Opet at Karnak, a house of the mysteries:

Southern wall: the good wind of the south; it is that which brings the Nile flood out of the cavern of the primaeval waters to inundate the earth with its all excellent products and supply food table with all good things for Osiris wenen-nefer, the justified.

The northern wall: The good wind of the north whose name is Kheb. The north wind of life, the breath that causes fields to rest, makes excellent the primaeval waters on earth and gives the breath of life to the nose of Osiris who is in the midst of Thebes.

The western wall: The good wind of the west, it is that which brings about the pouring down of the Nile flood of the sky, to make bright the land with plants, and bring into existence all the flowers for Osiris wenenen-nefer, the king of the gods, and isis the great, the god's mother and lady of all the gods.

The eastern wall: The good wind of the east: it is Osiris who daily begotten within the netherworld, It lifts up your ba to the sky together with the stars, Osiris wenen-nefer, the king of the gods.

Blue Magick Bath Oil

So, as you gather by now, blue magick represents the season of abundance, expansion, luxury and magic. We have magic all year round, but there is something very special in the depth and clarity of the endless shades of blue. One can dedicate all Wednesdays (Mercury/Thoth day) of the season for a ritual appreciation of the blue magick by inhaling the scent of blue magick and uttering the spell before inhalation or getting in the bath.

Blue magick spell

(Thoth Says)

Take a deep breath and inhale the beautiful, sweet aroma of Mercury Day. This will help attune you to the expansive energies and vibrations of Blue magick; leading you to discover hidden gems in the depths of the sea and brilliantly glowing crystals in the night sky.

In a little bowl mix -

1 tablespoon sea or Epsom salt/powdered milk/almond oil
A couple of Blue lotus dried flowers
A tablespoon full of dry chamomile flowers
1 drop of pure Jasmine essential oil
2 drops of pure frankincense essential oil
3 drops of pure bergamot essential oil
Say the spell while inhaling the oil blend before adding it to the bath, get in the bath and relax into the abundance and expansive qualities of the scent.

18. Black Magick Halloween/Samhain

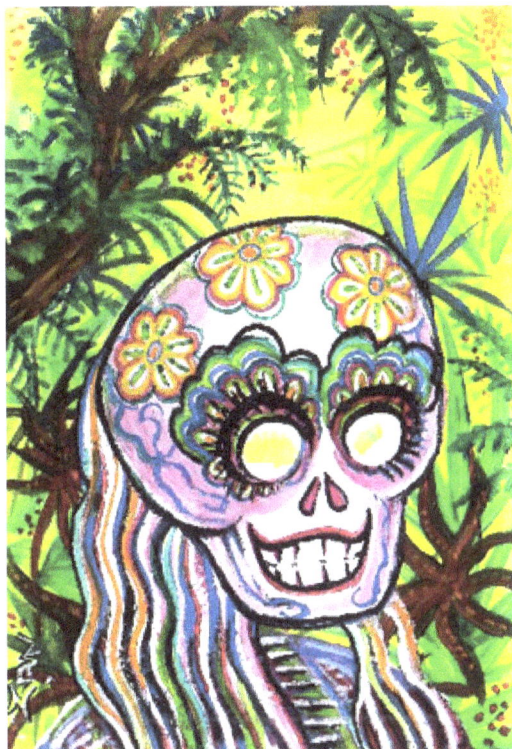

"Santa Muerte" by Jan Fries

October brings with it change. Autumn has arrived, and the harvest is behind us. We are now immersed in the 'darker half of the year', a period halfway between the Autumnal Equinox and Winter Solstice. This chapter of the annual cycle can be likened to Kali's dark sequence of the lunar month.

On the ancient Celtic festival Samhain, the new year is welcomed and the harvest season comes to a close to signal the start of winter - an era that was thought to represent death. Ancient Celts believed that on this special night, the divide between those alive and those who had passed away temporarily disappeared and the spirits of deceased ancestors could make contact. It is widely accepted that the Celtic festival of Samhain has had a strong influence on many Halloween traditions. Some believe that the early Church further developed it, Christianizing it as All Hallow's Day and its eve. On this day, people believed that the souls of those who passed away were trying to enter their homes, so they disguised themselves in costumes or lit bonfires to ward them off.

Samhain or Halloween, whichever you prefer to call it, marks the start of the Black Magick season which is probably the best time of the year to connect and pay homage to our ancestors. Though it may be challenging for some to bestow respect on those from their lineage, the concept of an ancestor can be broadened to encompass all that pre-dated us. Whatever his/her bloodline or traditions, ensure you honour them with proper respect and knowledge of their history on this Black Magick night.

The Black Magick season is significant for me, as it provides an opportunity to interact with our guardians and ancestors beyond the veil. It is also a moment to re-establish the promises we made in the past and those that are yet to come.

A few days before the black magick ritual I got a call from one of my coven's key members, telling me he won't be coming. I was gutted. G. is a very talented and sensitive young witch. He has a special gift, a unique way with words that got him the title "Spell Master". But sometimes words are not enough to cross the big gaping void in our hearts, and no spell seems to be effective when your days turn to one long night. G. has taken a break from everyday life and gone on a personal journey exploring the edges and depths of the Dark Night of the Soul. Those who have undertaken the dark journey of self-reflection before are very familiar with its consequences; we can only be present and provide comfort, lend an ear when wanted, and never pass judgement.

One aspect of black magic that is less talked about is the process of growth and regeneration which gives life. Solve et Coagula refers to the destruction needed before being able to construct something stronger and more useful than before.

Reflecting on the notion of Solve a Coagula got me thinking about the ancient Egyptian Osiris myth. According to Plutarch, Set conspires with seventy-two unseen allies to deceive Osiris. Set has a chest crafted to fit his exact size and at the banquet offers to give it away as a prize for whoever is capable of lying inside it. Those present were eager to try, yet none could fit except Osiris. When he laid down in the chest, Set and his associates slammed the lid shut, sealed it tightly, and cast it out into the river Nile. It journeyed far out into the sea, eventually reaching Byblos where a tree grew around it encasing Osiris's body within. The king of Byblos had the tree cut down and made into a pillar for his palace, with the chest containing Osiris' body still within. Isis had to extract it, but Set then stole it and dismembered the corpse. She gathered and buried each fragment except the penis, which was swallowed by a fish in the river; she used her magic to reconstruct it instead. Egyptian texts tell a different story, however, and in them the penis of Osiris is still intact.

I've long been perplexed by the story of Set slaying Osiris, dismembering him and discarding his phallus into the Nile.

It's clear that this act of aggression between the two brothers is about something more than just a territorial or marital dispute. What hidden symbolism could be behind this? One day, while working on a perfume blend for the black magick season, it dawned on me.

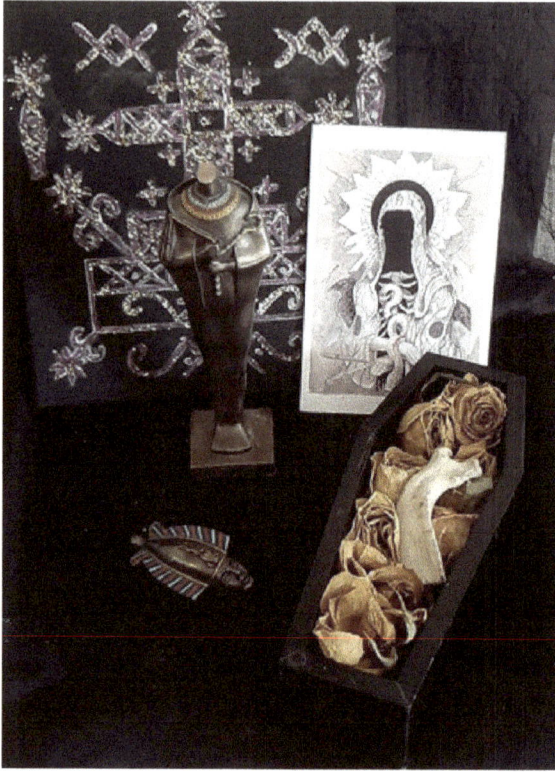

The river Nile is the life source of all of Egypt. The phallus is the symbol of life, procreation, and regeneration. By throwing it into the river, Set makes sure that the life force of the river will never cease or dry out. Ra's grandsons, Set and Osiris, form a sacred triad with their grandfather. To secure Ra's life, both brothers had to make a great sacrifice - Osiris by being slain by his brother Set; Set in turn was exiled for murdering his sibling. The river Nile is featured in the Amduat, where Osiris's phallus (the symbol of life and regeneration) helps keep Ra's vitality charged during his nocturnal voyage through the underworld.

It can certainly be argued that the first death of Osiris, drowning in a coffin, had an ambiguous significance within Egyptian culture. After all, the gift of a coffin was viewed as a way to grant immortality. Consequently, his later death by dismemberment may also have been interpreted with considerable complexity. After all, why didn't Seth just kill Osiris without the subterfuge? Some say it is an initiation, perhaps a demonic one.

Solve et Coagula – The dissolution of both brothers helps to uphold balance and ensure the preservation of Ra's might as well as that of the land's population and its environment.

Osiris's Dream Oil

The essential oils I used to create Osiris' Dream Perfume oil open a doorway of communication, enabling us to access our ancestors or look deeper into the underworld and the Amduat.

Vetiver, Galbanum, Clary sage, Elemi, Labdanum, Vervain. The use of vervain-Verbena officinalis, in this blend, was only for symbolic purposes - 2 drops of a tincture as a representative of the tears of Isis. The ancient Egyptians believed that Vervain grew out of the tears of the goddess Isis when she mourned the death of the god Osiris.

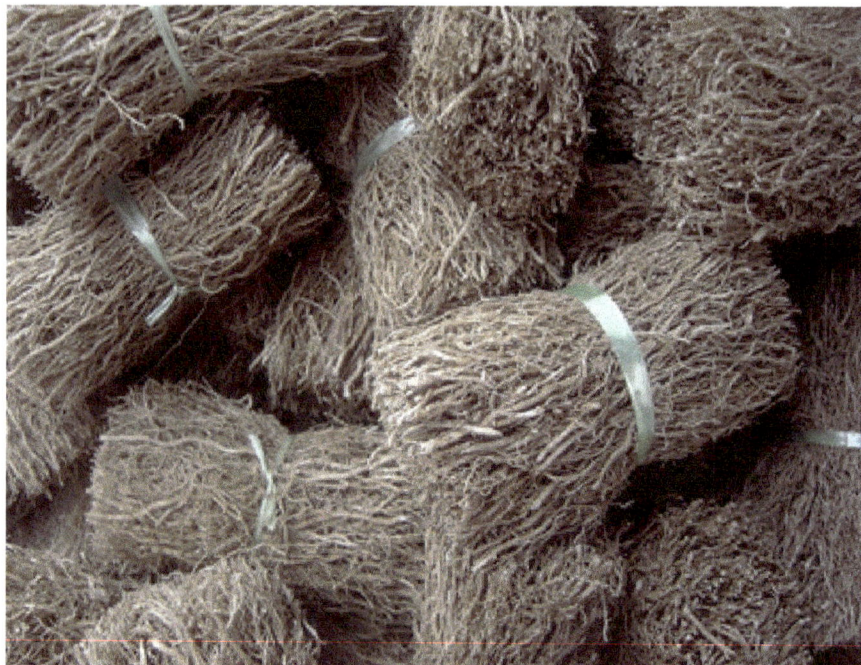

Vetiver, Vetiveria zizanoides

(Photo courtesy of wiki commons wikimedia.org)

Vetiver is a fragrant, perennial grass originating from South India, Indonesia and Sri Lanka. It has an impressive system of white rootlets which is used to produce essential oil through steam distillation; the process involves washing, chopping, drying and soaking the roots.

This dark brown to amber-coloured oil emits a unique aroma of smokiness, sweetness and an earthy, woody essence - just like the smell of the earth. Its cool and moist energy brings a sense of tranquillity yet invigorates us. It stimulates our circulation, helping to alleviate muscular pain and reduce recovery time for wounds. In India and Sri Lanka, the essence is known as the 'oil of tranquillity' which suggests its qualities to restore and calm an hyperactive mind.

I recall the first time I caught a whiff of Vetiver in my Introduction to Essential Oils course. Its powerful, soil-like aroma immediately registered with my sense of smell. I felt like I'd been pulled down through a dark and cold subterranean vortex of time and space. The aroma around me consumed my entire being and I became one with the heart of the geosphere, reconnecting with the roots of mother earth and restoring my connection to her, uniting my own beating heart with her own steady rhythm.

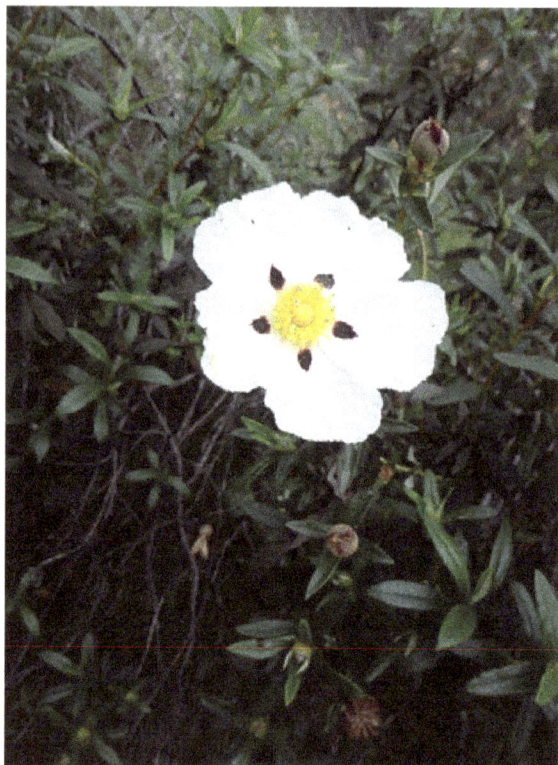

Labdanum, Cistus ladaniferus

(Photo courtesy of wiki commons wikimedia.org)

Labdanum is a small, fragrant shrub growing up to 3 metres high. Its lance-shaped leaves are indicative of the Mediterranean and Middle Eastern regions from which it originates. The dark brown gum-like oleoresin is obtained by boiling the plant material in water. Being a natural product, solvent extraction is used to produce the resin, while steam distillation from the crude gum, absolute or leaves/twigs enables the extraction of essential oil from this plant.

The dark sticky resinoid substance has a rich, sweet, balsamic, vanilla-like fragrance and can be used as a substitute for Ambergris. Labdanum was probably one of the earliest aromatic substances used in pharmacology and perfumery. The gum was used for catarrh, coughs and bronchitis symptoms, and also used for diarrhoea and to promote menstruation. Externally it was used in plasters and was one of the ingredients in beauty lotions of the women of the ancient world as a treatment for wrinkles and a nourishment for mature skin. The warm sweet slightly musty fragrance invokes within us the seeds of spiritual devotion and prayer and allows us to breathe calmly and deeply while meditating and reflecting.

I've already discussed the qualities of Galbanum, Elemi and Clary sage in earlier chapters. Still, just a little reminder, Galbanum is our gate opener, the psychopomp. The pungent herb-like scent of galbanum teleports us immediately into the musty darkness of the Tunnels of Set (check out Kenneth Grant's *Nightside of Eden*) that leads to the worlds beyond.

When our noses get used to the tunnels' mouldy dampness, we can detect a hint of the sweet, nutty-herbaceous scent of Clary sage. As its name suggests, Clary is the oil of clarity, clear thinking and clear visions, and this specific blend of oils will also promote clarity of communication. Next comes the heady fresh, balsamic-spicy odour of Elemi that brings with it a deeper insight and spiritual-psychedelic experience.

Having stepped through the portal deep into the heart of the earth's labyrinth, we can no longer deny the steady beat of Vetiver's signature scent – smoky, sweet and earthy - restoring our equilibrium and reminding us that regeneration, growth and birth all begin in this dark, mysterious place. As we delve further into the ground, the only scent detected is the rich, balsamic aroma of labdanum that lingered at the gateways of the hidden subterranean chamber. Its sweet vanilla-like fragrance evokes ancient memories of the obscure ceremonies carried out by Amun's priests, the Opening of The Mouth ritual, and breathing Ka back to Osiris.

Creating Osiris's dream perfume oil took me on an unusual voyage into the depths of my subconscious. Although I still don't have a complete grasp of the enigma of Osiris, making the oil through the month helped me to gain some understanding of his story.

While creating a perfume oil, I surround myself with the specific oils that will go into the blend and smell them all day long. I'll put a drop on a fragrance test paper and sniff it, mix a single essential oil in some carrier oil and rub it onto my wrists and under my nose. I'll put a few drops in the diffuser and in the bath. Once the blend is complete, I test its potency by rubbing a little of the perfume oil under my nose, wrists and behind my (and Mogg's) ears just before I go to bed.

Throughout the month of Osiris (see table of the Egyptian months at the end of the chapter), I used Osiris' dream perfume oil. I was inclined to name it Black Magick Perfume Oil, which fit perfectly with the time of year and forthcoming Black Sabbat. However, soon after applying it, I noticed how it affected my dreams.

My dreams descended into darker depths, full of ritualistic symbols and elements. Some nights I felt like I was exploring the shadowy tunnels of Set, with fierce demons at my heels. On other nights, I was led to a secret chamber to witness a complex ritual of the priests of Amun. During that full month, these dreams were extremely vivid and felt incredibly authentic. Some nights I woke up startled and confused, scared to go back to sleep. Most mornings I woke up very tired and exhausted as if I was engaged in some serious physical activity during the night.

It didn't take long for me to realise the potency of the perfume and its part as the key to Osiris's Dream realm so I renamed it accordingly.

Gods of Lunar Year					
Month	Neter	Name	Hieroglyph		
(Jul)	Thoth	Thoth	*dhwty*		
1 (Jul-Aug)	Seth	Tekhy	*thy*		
2 (Aug - Sep)	Min	Phaophi	*p n jpt*	Akhet (inundation)	
3 (Sep - Oct)	Hathor	Athyr	*Hwt-hr*		
4 (Oct-Nov)	Sokar	Choiak	*k3 hr k3*		
5 (Nov - Dec)	Neith	Tyby	*t3 ᶜbt*		
6 (Dec - Jan)	Nuit	Mechir	*mhyr*	Peret (planting)	
7 (Jan-Feb)	Anubis	Pharmenoth	*p n jmn htp*		
8 (Feb - Mar)	Renenutet	Pharmuthi	*p n rnwtt*		
9 (Mar - Apr)	Khonsu	Pachon	*Hnsw*		
10 (Apr -	Horus	Payni	*Hnt-hty*	Shemu (harvest)	
11 (May -	Ipet	Epiphi	*ᶜlpt*		
12 (Jun - Jul)	Ra	Mesore	*mswt rᶜ*		

An extra or intercalary or epagomenal month of Thoth is
added to the lunar calendar every two to three years to
keep it synchronized with the seasons.

Overcoming Apep

Part of my day job is reading and editing books, recently I was preparing the ebook edition of Seth & The Two Ways (Morgan 2019). Reading Appendix 2 – Book(s) of Overthrowing Apep (Bremner Rhind Papyrus 3), a papyrus found in Thebes (in Upper Egypt), thought to be from the tomb of a priest of the Ptolemaic period, with intense and formidable curses inside. In order to complete the editing task, I had to read all nine books in one sitting.

As I made my way through the texts, I became increasingly disturbed. The words of the books seemed to come alive as if they were being uttered directly at me. This feeling was incredibly unsettling and left me greatly troubled. By the time I reached book three, the oppressive despair had shifted to something else – an emotion that was difficult to pinpoint.

As I went through books three and four, a powerful sensation flooded my body, causing a surge of energy to course up and down my spine – as if some sort of potent circle had formed around me. At the beginning of book five, The Book of Knowing The Creation Of Ra And Of Overthrowing Apep, I was surrounded by an aura of power, giving me a feeling of security and strength. I could sense something significant was about to come.

By the time I finished reading book six, I had an insight into the nature of cursing and the importance of the god Seth in Egyptian Cosmology and its pantheons.

The ninth book vibrates the victorious rhythms of mission accomplished, the priest ferried through the most horrendous and atrocious curses, his spirit never failing, his heart never broken, his body fully charged with the primaeval power of the ancient serpent that vibrates with the secrets of creation. He is one with the Dark Lord, with the Red God, with the Black power of the North, he is ready to take on the ancient worm.

By the time I finished reading the ninth book, I felt powerful, strong, determined, and mighty. I was ready to slay a dragon.

Most of the curses and "grimoires" we are familiar with are working on a very specific psychological level – earthy and primal, to intimidate and bully a person, in the most extreme and influential ways, to make them believe they are cursed. As we know, this power is indisputable and when a person believes in something, it can be nearly impossible to argue with them or to change their minds.

This type of cursing is directed straight to the emotional centre, resonating with the lower and earthly vibrations to cause fear and upheaval in the lives of the 'victim'. On the other hand, the person who does the cursing is as much trapped in the emotional realm of aggression and intimidation as the target is.

To curse an awesome and primaeval power such as Apep, the priest who conducted the ritual, needed to be as strong and as powerful as Apep, probably stronger.

I have come to believe that the Book(s) of Overthrowing Apep was meant to be read and performed as one ritual without a break. Like many other Egyptian texts, the Bremner Rhind Papyrus 3 is a text that takes us on a journey of becoming. The priest or priests build up their mental and physical resilience by vibrating those hostile words, channelling the power and assimilating them into themselves, transforming those nine books of curses into a mighty weapon of protection and strength.

I mentioned above how these texts were probably found in the tomb of a priest. They were included as part of the funeral rites and preparation for the underworld or night journey. Whichever way one looks at it, one can't avoid the awareness that Apep is eternal, bornless and cannot be killed. This realisation could cause a psychological battle in the mind of the priest, leading to doubts, despair and resentment of his beliefs, and losing their ability to perform their roles properly in the temple. By turning the tables and learning the secrets powers of the curse, the priest acquires a tool of power, channelling those of the cursed one onto himself, freeing himself from the mundane state of existence, transforming and attuning his mind into the cosmic rhythm of the eternal.

Being equipped with such a papyrus, with such a powerful curse, in the tomb on your final journey, would be like the ultimate insurance policy against the immense forces of Apep the eternal, to protect his "soul" (Ba, Ka, Akh) on the final journey.

The Names Of Apep

Which Shall Have No Existence

Book nine is like a repetitive mantra to be chanted and written on papyrus and to be burned in the fire. In the mantra, the name of Apep is repeated twenty-nine times! Each repetition is written with one of his terrible and horrific powerful characteristics, for instance - (21) Apep Kher Amam (Apep, The Fallen, The Devourer) (25) Apep Kher Kenemmti (Apep, The Fallen, The Dark One) (28) Apep Kher Sekhem-her (Apep, The Fallen, The Potent of Glance). Ostensibly it looks as if the priest is chanting and writing a very fierce curse. From my personal experience with mantra chantings, I can say that the more you repeat the same word, vowel or seed mantra, the more you can actually feel the energy gathering, charging and vibrating around and within you. You are becoming one with the rhythm, like the physical vessel of the mantra vibrations. The repetition of Apep's name is the way in which the priest channels and charges the power into himself.

According to the instructions on the Abydos Temple walls, the daily temple ritual was performed three times a day. Based on information from Temple Ritual at Abydos by Rosalie David (2016), before entering the temple, the priests had to purify themselves in the water basins, the sacred lake or any other convenient pure water source. Weapons must be left outside the temple and only then can they approach the shrine door.

They open that door while saying: "I remove the finger of Seth from the Eye of Horus" stepping into the shrine and looking at the God, saying whatever comes into their mind as a greeting. Perhaps something like this: "Be not unaware of me (Ra), If you know me, I will know you". They move into the shrine and stand before the altar and clean away any debris, tidy the place, light the fire and anointed all the deities statues and figurines with the daily perfume and made an offering of food etc saying: "Hetep di nesew asir neb djedu neter Aa neb Abdu" Which was the standard offering formula in Egyptian rites and can be adapted to any deity. Once all this was done, the priest positioned himself in front of the offering table and started to read the Book(s) of Overthrowing Apep, building up the energy to the triumphant crescendo of the chanting the words of book nine – The Names Of Apep Which Shall Have No Existence, finishing the rite by throwing a wax image into the purifying flames of the temple fire.

One can almost see the rite taking place and the vibrations of the chants resonating within the temple. Now imagine how it would feel to visit that temple when the ritual of Overthrowing Apep has been performed a myriad times, since the Middle Kingdom when its existence was first recorded. For the uninitiated and the laymen, the temples in which this

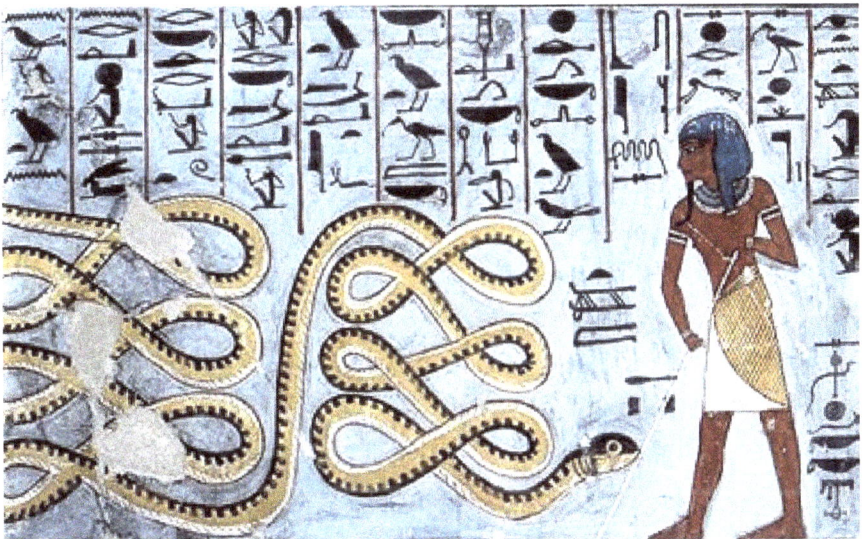

Apep being warded off by a deity.
Tomb of pharaoh Ramses I. Thebes West, near 1307 BC.

(Photo courtesy of wiki commons wikimedia.org)

rite has been regularly performed must have been the most forbidding and eerie of places, haunted by wild-eyed priests. For the cult and its initiates, this was a place of power, a place to immerse yourself and to be charged with the endless *baraka* of the eternal one.

The Sethian myth is established on the sacred triad: Ra, Seth & Apophis, none could exist without the others. It is the battle dance of creation, one dies, another must kill and one must shine.

19. Valediction

Since antiquity, we have followed the changes of the seasons and the rhythms of the moon. Using the methods outlined in this book, you can reach new realms of awareness, cosmic knowledge, mystic synchronizations and sensory pleasure. The first section of the book covers the Kala cycle, emphasizing both its dark/Kali and light/Shakti aspects. The second part examines the witches eight sabbats in depth.

You can enter the Aromagick voyage at any time during the Lunar cycle. Each Kala serves as a portal or a key to access the power of that special day. This alignment with corresponding lunar energies is more effortless when experienced during the 4 cardinal Kalas which are:

Kameswari – new moon
Duti/Tavrita – first quarter
Amrita/Kali – full moon
Ugra/Ugraprabha – last quarter

Note: It is hard to distinguish between Mudra and Mita with one's naked eye when Kameswari arrives with the initial illumination of the month. I believe that this is the optimal time to align oneself with Lunar energies.

In chapter 11 I wrote of how the Ancient Romans linked Chronos with Saturn, a deity in their own pantheon. Chronos was one of three gods that represented the idea of time within Greek mythology, alongside Aion and Kairos. The lunar cycle is governed by the Timelord Kairos, which symbolises opportunistic time - moments when action must be taken to move forward. The 8 witches' sabbats and each Kala offer us the chance to unravel the enigmas of time. As we progress on our journey, we come to understand that the wheel of the year and the lunar cycles are not separate entities, but rather intertwined in a never-ending spiral. This spiral continues to deepen and refine us, making us capable of exerting mastery over time, like Timelords.

A ritual bath will facilitate a perfect experience of psychological, spiritual and mysticism. Using pure essential oils and high-quality fragrances will provide the full experience and benefits. If you are new to Aromatherapy and blending essential oils, I highly recommend you adhere to the guidance given at the end of chapter 14. To use a single essential oil in a bath, 7-10 drops should suffice; anything more than 15 drops should be avoided. Essential oils and water do not mix, so to get the most out of their properties a conductor such as sea or Epsom salts, milk powder or vegetable oil must be included to enable the essential oils molecules to enter the water. Therefore, for optimal results when using essential oils in your ritual bath or any other type of bath, these carriers should be implemented.

What to do if you don't have a bath but still want to use essential oils?

An easy way to connect with the spirit of the essential oil is to open up the bottle and take in its aroma during your ritual when focusing internally or meditating. Additionally, if you intuitively feel "called" by the oil you can do so at any time.

Initiation oils are a good way to connect with their spirit and/or energies, with the Kalas or any one of the 8 witches' sabbats. If you want to make your own initiation oil, use a carrier oil like almond (it barely has a scent, unlike olive oil which has an intense aroma and can affect the final smell) or any other vegetable oil of your choice will do. A simple recipe involves combining 5 drops of essential oil with one tablespoon of vegetable oil.

More advanced recipes will require some basic knowledge of aromatherapy.

Creating the Aromagick perfume oils was part of the process of writing this book, every dream, insight and understanding of the nature of the Kalas and the 8 colours of magick was the result of weeks, sometimes months, meditating with different essential oils and fragrances, to create the essence that will capture my understanding of each Kala, colour and Sabbat. Each blend has a unique quality of evoking within us the essence of the spirits and energies mentioned above. It may not be possible for the reader to duplicate this part of the magick for themselves, so I'm making available the fruits of my own efforts as a collection.

The Aromagick perfume oil collection offers a completely transformative experience of the aromas of the witches' sabbats or any of the Kalas discussed in this book. This set includes eight bottles of magick in all the colours, as well as two additional perfume bottles of different Kalas. All are presented beautifully in a red case.

A diffuser is another way to enjoy the benefits of essential oils if you don't have access to a bath. Electric diffusers can be used for this purpose, as they convert fragrance or essential oil into a gentle mist that spreads its aroma throughout the surrounding area. Using a diffuser during a ritual is an excellent way of immediately setting the atmosphere. The number of drops required for the diffuser will depend on the size of your room.

Every oil and perfume blend mentioned in this book has the potential to influence our memories, feelings and dreams. To intensify your dream quality and experience, I suggest applying perfume oil to the pulse points behind your ears, on your wrists and under your nose, before bed. A specially designed diffuser blend can also be used if you wish to evoke lucid dreaming while asleep.

The Aromagick collection is designed to provide a gateway into the realm of dreams. Intermediate and advanced dreamers alike can access the temples within their subconscious. Each perfume serves as a key, unlocking secret doors of the mind.

I believe that with the first inhalation, scents, aromas and fragrances can link us to the divine. My personal experiences described here in the book, mirror the links and connections we all can make with our subconsciousness and other realms, using our olfactory senses. The essential oils I chose to write about have a scentual signature that evokes specific memories, of lost empires and ancient lands, of gods and goddesses, black magick, dragons and demons. Those occult memories will haunt our dreams, as messengers from other times and outer spaces.

I believe with one breath that scents, aromas and fragrances bring us closer to the divine. Through my own experiences documented in this book, it is possible to unlock connections and gain access to other realms using smell alone. These vibrant recollections reach far beyond our mortal realm, to awaken visions in our dreams; messages from different times and outer space.

Time is Kali
Space is Lalita

The Devi Prayer

Maa Amba Lalita Devi, Parashakti Sundari
Namastasyai Namastasyai Namastasyai Namo Namah

Maa Amba Lalita Devi, Mahamaye Mangale
Namastasyai Namastasyai Namastasyai Namo Namah

Maa Amba Lalita Devi, Mahakali Bhairavi
Namastasyai Namastasyai Namastasyai Namo Namah

Maa Amba Lalita Devi, Mahalakshmi Vaishnavi
Namastasyai Namastasyai Namastasyai Namo Namah

Maa Amba Lalita Devi, Ma Sarasvati Brahmi
Namastasyai Namastasyai Namastasyai Namo Namah

Maa Amba Lalita Devi, Durga Devi Shankari
Namastasyai Namastasyai Namastasyai Namo Namah

Maa Amba Lalita Devi, Uma Parvati Shive
Namastasyai Namastasyai Namastasyai Namo Namah

Maa Amba Lalita Devi, Ma Bhavani Ambike
Namastasyai Namastasyai Namastasyai Namo Namah

Maa Amba Lalita Devi, Annapurna Lakshmi Ma
Namastasyai Namastasyai Namastasyai Namo Namah

Maa Amba Lalita Devi, Kamala Katyayani
Namastasyai Namastasyai Namastasyai Namo Namah

Maa Amba Lalita Devi, Tvam Brahmani Gayatri
Namastasyai Namastasyai Namastasyai Namo Namah

Maa Amba Lalita Devi, Tvam Tripura Sundari
Namastasyai Namastasyai Namastasyai Namo Namah

Maa Amba Lalita Devi, Mata Bhuvaneshvari

Namastasyai Namastasyai Namastasyai Namo Namah

Maa Amba Lalita Devi, Tvam Raja Rajeshvari
Namastasyai Namastasyai Namastasyai Namo Namah

Maa Amba Lalita Devi, Bhagavati Bhargavi
Namastasyai Namastasyai Namastasyai Namo Namah

Maa Amba Lalita Devi, Parabhakti Varade
Namastasyai Namastasyai Namastasyai Namo Namah

Maa Amba Lalita Devi, Maya Vishvamohini
Namastasyai Namastasyai Namastasyai Namo Namah

Maa Amba Lalita Devi, Ishvari Narayani
Namastasyai Namastasyai Namastasyai Namo Namah

Maa Amba Lalita Devi, Nitya Parameshvari
Namastasyai Namastasyai Namastasyai Namo Namah

Maa Amba Lalita Devi, Jagadambe Janani
Namastasyai Namastasyai Namastasyai Namo Namah

Maa Amba Lalita Devi, Tvam Anandasagari
Namastasyai Namastasyai Namastasyai Namo Namah

Sarva Mangala Mangalye
Shive Sarvartha Sadhike
Sharanye Tryambake Devi
Narayani Namostute
Narayani Namostute
Narayani Namostute
Om Shanti Shanti Shantihi

Aromagick perfume & bath oil collection

The Eight Colours of Magick*:

Octarine magic

Green magic

Orange magic

Purple magic

Yellow magic

Red magic

Blue magic

Black magic

* The 8 magicks can be bought as a complete set or as individual items.

The Kalas:

Kameswari

Nityaklinna

Shivaduti

Lalita

Kali

Kulla

Kurukulla

Ugra

Mudra

Mita

Mahahkali

Lunar:

Dark moon

New moon

First quarter

Full moon

Last quarter

Deities:

Pan – K23

Baphomet

Osiris's dream

Orders via mandrake.uk.net

Bibliography

Ashley, Elizabeth (2016) *Helichrysum For The Wound That Will Not Heal*. IP.

Avalon, Arthur (1974) *The Serpent Power*. Dover.

Carroll, Peter J. (1987) *Liber Null & Psychonaut*. Weiser.

Carroll, Peter J. (1992) *Liber Kaos*. Weiser.

Crowley, Aleister (2004) *Liber Al vel Legis*. Red Wheel/Weiser.

Crowley, Aleister (1994) "Liber Resh vel Helios" pp. 645-646 in *Magick, Liber ABA*, Weiser.

Crowley, Aleister (1983) *The Book of Thoth*. U.S. Games Systems.

Crowley, Aleister (1989) *The Confessions of Aleister Crowley*. Edited by Symonds John & Kenneth Grant. Arkana.

Crowley, Aleister (1977) *The Qabalah of Aleister Crowley*. Weiser.

Cunningham, Scott (1997) *Magical Aromatherapy*. Llewellyn.

Danielou, Alain (1991) *The Myths and Gods of India*. Inner Traditions.

David, A. Rosalie (2016) *Temple Ritual at Abydos*. London, . Print.

Desikachar, T.K.V. (1999) *The Heart of Yoga*. Inner Traditions.

Drummond, Bill and Jimmy Cauty (2017) *2023: A Trilogy by The Justified Ancient of Mu Mu*. Faber and Faber.

Farber, Phillip H. (2010) *The Great Purple Hoo-Ha*. Mandrake.

Grant, Kenneth (1973) *Aleister Crowley and The Hidden God*. Muller.

Grant, Kenneth (1977) *Nightside of Eden*. Muller.

Grant, Kenneth (1980) *Outside the Circles of Time*. Muller

Hornung, Erik, and David Lorton. *History of Ancient Egypt : An Introduction*. Ithaca, N.Y., 1999. Print.

Kelly, Michael (2011) *Dragonscales*. IP

Kelly, Michael (2020) *The Satanic Dragon*. IP.

Lawless, Julia (1995) *The Illustrated Encyclopedia of Essential Oils: The Complete Guide to the Use of Oils in Aromatherapy and Herbalism* Illustrated Encyclopedia

Series. Element

Le Guin, Ursula K. (2016) *Earthsea*. Penguin.

MacRae, George W. "The Thunder, Perfect Mind" published in *Nag Hammadi Codices* V, 2-5 and VI with Papyrus Berolinensis 8502, 1 and 4. Parrott, Alexander, editor. Brill Academic Publishers. (1979) Leiden; Boston : BRILL 1 online resource.

Magee, Mike (2022) *Kali Magic*. Twisted Trunk.

Malphas (2009) *The Black Ship*. Sirius Ink.

Mastros, Sara L. (2021) *The Big Book of Magical Incense*. Weiser.

Mojay, Gabriel (1999) *Aromatherapy for Healing the Spirit*. Gaia.

Morgan, Mogg (2019) *Seth & The Two Ways*. Mandrake.

Morgan, Mogg (2021) *Egyptian Magick*. Mandrake.

Morgan, Mogg (2022) *Aleister Crowley & Thelemic Magick*. Mandrake.

Peters, Gregory (2022) *Yogini Magic*. Falcon.

Power, John (2002) *The NU Tantras of the Uttarakaulas*. Mandrake.

Pratchett, Terry (1988) *The Colour of Magic*. Corgi.

Robbins, Tom (2019) *Jitterbug Perfume*. No Exit Press.

Roy, Michael (May 23, 2020). "The Three Greek Gods of Time." https://medium.com/minute-mythology/the-three-greek-gods-of-time-60f236ae16e9

Shivashakti.com (Mike Magee) "The Fifteen Nityas" : shivashakti.com/nitya

Shulke, Daniel (2000) *Ars Philtron*. XOANON.

Sri Lalita Sahsranama (1996) *The Thousand Names of the Divine Mother*. Ammachi.

Vayne, Julian & Steve Dee (2014) *Chaos Craft*. IP.

Walsh, Coleen "What the Nose Knows" - *The Harvard Gazette, Science & Technology*, online journal accessed 27/2/2020

Warner, Felicity (2018) *Sacred Oils*. Hay House.

Essential Oils in this book

Index

www.ingramcontent.com/pod-product-compliance
Lightning Source LLC
Chambersburg PA
CBHW050808270326
41926CB00026B/4631